For everyone involved in Shared Lives
and Homeshare.

And for Katie, Django and Louis who share their
lives with me.

A NEW HEALTH AND CARE SYSTEM

Escaping the invisible asylum

Alex Fox

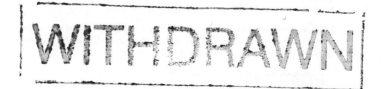

First published in Great Britain in 2018 by

Policy Press
University of Bristol
1-9 Old Park Hill
Bristol BS2 8BB
UK
t: +44 (0)117 954 5940
e: pp-info@bristol.ac.uk
www.policypress.co.uk

North American office:
Policy Press
c/o The University of Chicago Press
1427 East 60th Street
Chicago, IL 60637, USA
t: +1 773 702 7700
f: +1 773-702-9756
e:sales@press.uchicago.edu
www.press.uchicago.edu

British Library Cataloguing in Publication Data
A catalogue record for this book is available from the British Library.

Library of Congress Cataloging-in-Publication Data
A catalog record for this book has been requested.

ISBN 978-1-4473-4167-3 (paperback)
ISBN 978-1-4473-4175-8 (ePub)
ISBN 978-1-4473-4176-5 (Kindle)
ISBN 978-1-4473-4174-1(ePDF)

Cover design by Policy Press
Front cover: image kindly supplied by PicFair
Printed and bound in Great Britain by Clays Ltd, St Ives plc
Policy Press uses environmentally responsible print partners

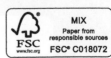

MIX
Paper from
responsible sources
FSC® C018072

Contents

Acknowledgements

I would like to thank everyone who has been involved in Shared Lives, Homeshare and the other approaches I make reference to in this book: their mostly untold stories form the basis of the ideas I attempt to present here. I would particularly like to thank my colleagues at Shared Lives Plus, as well as Sian Lockwood OBE and her colleagues at Community Catalysts, for their inspiring work. There are of course countless other approaches which I either have not come across or couldn't find space for – my apologies. Many people kindly gave permission for their stories to be used: thank you. Some names and other details have been changed.

I'm grateful to the following people who have in different ways given me help, insight or inspiration: my parents, Professor Chris Fox, Vickie Cammack, Al Etmanski, Philipa Bragman and the team at CHANGE, Dame Philippa Russell DBE, Ralph Broad, Sam Clark, Martin Routledge, Anna McEwen, Clenton Farquharson MBE, Professor Saul Becker, Des Benjamin, Matthew Taylor, Halima Khan, Richard Jones CBE.

I could not have written this book without the wisdom and support of my partner Katie.

All errors and omissions are my own.

Prologue

As early as the 14th century, a small town called Geel in Belgium was visited by mentally ill pilgrims from across Europe. Geel houses a shrine to St Dymphna, the patron saint of mental illness. Rather than building an asylum outside of the city walls, the medieval town organised itself into a 'boarding out' system which still exists today, in which people were supported in ordinary family homes. This early example of 'care in the community' recognised the ability of ordinary people to provide support to people who might more normally have been shunned and feared. Geel became a place which gave asylum rather than building them.

In the centuries that followed, few places followed Geel's example, but many asylums and institutions were built to keep disabled people, those with mental health problems, the sick and the old outside of our communities. In more recent history, most asylum, workhouse and long-stay hospital buildings have been closed and the services they housed moved into ordinary houses. Conversely, the work that took place in those buildings has become increasingly professionalised and further removed from what we expect ordinary people to be able to do. Despite these outward changes, many of the assumptions first rejected by the people of Geel centuries ago persist, invisibly but tenaciously, in the new 'community settings' of our health, care and other support services.

The people of medieval Geel chose a way of thinking about care for people who need long-term support which still seems both shockingly radical and entirely natural. They refused to see living as part of community as incompatible with either receiving or giving care. It is a way of thinking that has flickered in and out of the consciousness of those who seek to help others for seven centuries. I work for the charity that is charged with keeping alive that idea, which we now call 'Shared Lives' and which currently offers support, a home, and often love, to over 13,000 people across the UK.

Seven centuries later, it's an idea which may finally be about to have its day.

Introduction

The question of who is helped by government has for centuries been a question of who is included and excluded from their communities. Many would see government help as a safety net which cannot capture everyone, but needs to ensure that the most sick and poor do not fall outside society. But the origins of the welfare state lie equally in decisions about who to exclude from the tangible, local communities in which we live.

The first Poor Laws, in Tudor times, were mainly concerned with punishing the idle workless and sending them back to their place of origin to work. These parish–administered systems were subsumed by the national system of the New Poor Law in the 19th century, which established workhouses as a combined form of punishment and 'relief'. They removed paupers from the streets into institutions designed to be less attractive than the most menial of independent circumstances.

There had been lunatic asylums in Britain from the conversion of the Priory of the New Order of St Mary of Bethlem from a centre for alms collection in the 13th century, to a hospital and lunatic asylum in the 14th century, which gained notoriety as Bedlam. 'Madness' was mainly regarded as a domestic and parish issue, with only a small number of religious and charitable asylums, until the 1808 County Asylums Act empowered magistrates to build asylums in every county for 'pauper lunatics'. These captured (literally) a broad range of groups including those we would today label as having a mental illness, a learning disability or a substance misuse problem, but also people who were considered to have stepped outside of contemporary moral boundaries, such as unwed mothers (Brunton, 2004; Porter, 2006). The number of institutions and of people inside them grew into many tens of thousands by the 20th century. A medical model of mental illness was gradually introduced into the institutions, where it coexisted and became entwined with religious, criminal justice and charitable ideas.

Welfare legislation in the 20th century abolished the workhouse for healthy workless people, replacing it with largely financial assistance, and transferred responsibility for institutional care for the 'disabled, sick and aged' to local government and then, in 1948, to the National Assistance Board and the new National Health Service (NHS).

It's easy to read changes in long-term care since then as a gradual – if often painful and faltering – progression away from large institutions and towards support which takes place within 'the community'. Following countercultural revolutions in mental health care that started in the 1960s, long-stay hospitals for people with mental health problems have been closed, as have the largest and most visible institutions for people with learning disabilities or physical impairments.

But also in that period, the hospital has become the totemic symbol of healthcare, the large care home has remained and is on the rise as the default model of care for older people with high support needs, and the number of people with learning disabilities admitted into largely hidden 'special hospitals' grew and has proved resistant to reduction, despite the outcry caused by BBC's *Panorama* exposé of the Winterbourne View Assessment and Treatment Centre and subsequent high-profile 'improvement' programme. Meanwhile, in other parts of the public service world, prison sentences and populations grew, even as crime levels shrank and varieties of enforced labour are periodically resurrected as solutions to the 'idle poor'. As John Hills (2014) and others have argued, a distinction between the deserving and undeserving poor has been and is being 'hardwired' into welfare systems and the public consciousness.

So it is harder to find and see institutions, with their high walls and locked doors, but the language of public service assessment and eligibility is that of 'gateways' (with their 'gatekeepers'), 'thresholds' and 'pathways'. To enter our long-term health and care systems is to pass through an entrance which may open as rarely – and shut as resoundingly behind you – as any workhouse or asylum door.

In the health and care sectors there is wide consensus on the need to keep people from arriving at hospital gates and other forms of institutional care. But while ideas of prevention and early intervention are based on the belief that the boundaries can be redrawn, not erased, they themselves rest on familiar assumptions about the divide between community-based citizens and the subjects of service land, rather than removing that divide.

There was a period in the middle and late 20th century when visits to the hospital were comparatively rare and brief, as the NHS became adept at treating many diseases and most deaths in old age followed relatively short illnesses. But as the rise in life expectancy outpaces the rise in healthy life expectancy, now 15 million of us live with at least one long-term condition (including the majority of over-60s), and by 2018, nearly 3 million will live with three or more conditions (Department of Health, 2012), each the domain of a separate set of services and professionals. Most of us will care for at least one family member at some point in our lives; 6.5 million and rising at any one time. Dementia affects 850,000 people and millions of their relatives. As we become more mobile and less family- and community-rooted, new epidemics of poor wellbeing or mental health are growing, such as the epidemic of loneliness which sucks the joy from life for hundreds of thousands of older people, including 4 million who say the TV is their main source of company (Davidson and Rossall, 2014). Loneliness is shown to lead to poor physical as well as mental health, even increasing the risk of mortality (Holt-Lunstad et al, 2010). Medical advances are enabling most people with learning disabilities to outlive their parents for the first time, but the 'special' education system does not yet routinely enable them to enter adulthood as confident, socially connected full citizens.

What happens on the other side of the public service gateway has always contained much that we would consider undesirable and would prefer to ignore. For some early institutions, punishment or correction of their deviant inhabitants was deliberately built in. Later, the dehumanising effects of the 'total institution' (Goffman, 1961) ossified relationships between the keepers and the kept, with some institutions run for the employment of their staff, rather than for the benefit of their 'sub-human' inhabitants' (Foot, 2016). The 1960s saw physical institutions under concerted attack from radicals (R.D. Laing in the UK and Franco Basaglia in Italy, and the 'anti-psychiatrists') and the establishment: Enoch Powell, as Health Minister in 1961 talked famously of storming the defences of institutions which

> stand, isolated, majestic, imperious, brooded over by the gigantic water-tower and chimney combined, rising unmistakable and daunting out of the countryside – the asylums which our forefathers built with such immense solidity to express the notions of their day. Do not for a moment underestimate their powers of resistance to our assault. (Powell's speech to the Conservative Party conference, 1961)

Powell's ten-year plan to move care into the community took 20 to 30 years, but the most visible institutions were dismantled or repurposed during that time.

In recent decades, public service modernisation drew heavily from what were seen as the lessons of private-sector service industries, considered more dynamic and efficient by policy makers frustrated with the slow pace of change possible within long-established state services. The ethos of 'customer service' has made a positive impact on many brief service transactions. A 'customer' is likely to be treated with more courtesy and respect than a 'service user'. But the relationship between customer and supplier is a shallow and transactional one. The private sector has little track record of helping people to build and maintain relationships, sustain family life or become active in their community. For those using most health and care services, who are attempting to live well with a long-term – often lifelong – condition, spending lengthy spells inside institutionally organised buildings and systems continues to be an experience of living apart from the real life of family and community; of being a patient rather than a person; a customer rather than a citizen.

The people who find themselves with a long-term future inside service systems have historically been in a poor position to demand change. But more and more of us have extended personal or family experiences of living within service systems. Meanwhile, the disability rights, family carers and patient voice movements have made more visible those systems' limitations and failures and social media enables people to communicate their experience with the outside world. These demographic and cultural changes continued to accelerate as austerity bit and many services' staffing, quality and safety went into real decline. The language of 'customers', 'choice' and 'quality' only compounds the dissonance between what people hope their experience of support will be and the often bleak reality, while people working in those services find themselves the representatives of systems which can feel as inhuman to work in as to live in.

This amounts to a crisis in our perception of public services and the welfare state, as both the ingrained and the recently created problems within public services become harder for the general population to ignore. It also offers an opportunity to bring into full visibility both what is precious and what is pernicious within our long-term support services: the asylum they offer us when our wellbeing is threatened, and the asylums they can become if their grip is too unyielding.

The most innovative services now recognise that requiring entrants to surrender their passports and citizenship at the door is not only morally wrong but also self-defeating, if the goal is shared responsibility for long-term wellbeing. Rather than 'gatekeeping' dwindling resources and practising 'demand reduction', they are beginning to explore how they can build a new partnership with the people they support. This change requires services and the professionals who work within them to have clarity and confidence in what they can achieve, and realism and humility about what they cannot. It is that most elusive of service transformations: a 'culture change'. New ways of working alongside people rather than for them can be experienced as liberating by front-line professionals, even as they unsettle managers and decision makers. But it will not happen through only cultural means: it requires a fundamental shift of power, money and responsibility, without which more human and relational ways of working are crushed by short-term demands and risk-obsessed bureaucracies.

Some UK public services have been at the forefront of attempts to 'personalise' their work and are increasingly keen students of 'asset-based' community-building approaches developed in the US and elsewhere. The NHS talks increasingly of being 'patient centred' or even, 'person centred', ideas seemingly so self-evident that the need for their introduction says a lot about where this £120 billion system has been 'centred' previously. Yet, as a *Journal of Clinical Nursing* editorial noted, there is still no agreed definition of 'person centred' and most nurses (in common with many other care and health professionals) work 'in contexts and cultures that are inherently unsupportive of person-centredness' (Dewing and McCormack, 2016).

While there has been some progress in recognising that 'patients' and 'service users' are individuals and citizens, with unique life goals and the potential to take or at least share responsibility for reaching them, attempts to bring citizen-power into service design and management have been scarce and, usually, effectively suppressed or subverted by the power structures they challenge. Trust and faith in people in general, and in citizens with long-term support needs in particular, has been limited on the Right to selfish-gene beliefs in market forces and largely absent on the Left, which (despite its roots in mutuality and the cooperative movement) reserves its faith for the welfare state and post-Blair, has regarded 'consumerist' ideas of public service choice and individual budget control with suspicion.

This book is not an attack on services, an argument for small government, nor wishful thinking about the capacity of voluntary action. No solution offered in this book would justify further cuts to public service budgets, which have already been cut below the GDP proportions of comparable nations with increasingly visible results. Mainstream public services as they stand remain vital to protect us against the most dramatic of life's calamities. But even with adequate funding, they are by their nature incapable of fixing problems, such as loneliness, which are rooted in our changing relationships with others. Community groups, meanwhile (typically small, patchy in coverage and fragile) are set up to provide the kinds of support which most closely resemble what communities do 'naturally', which doesn't generally include the intensive and regular personal care of strangers.

Proponents of the Third Way (Giddens, 1998) set out an approach to public services which would remove the fossilised bureaucracies of traditional public services, replacing them with the pragmatism that they saw in the more dynamic private sector, driven by feedback, data and choice. Reforms that followed under Blair, however, accepted the underlying power differentials between people who live and work in services, and those who run and own them, instead putting faith in the ability of well-motivated and skilled managers, leaders and entrepreneurs to harness market forces and innovation for the common good. Public service leaders wrestled with how services could achieve outcomes, but did not enable people to define those outcomes for themselves. Theirs was a problem-solving mentality which, coupled with significant investment, fixed some failing services, but often slipped into the fallacy that people's lives can also be fixable.

Throughout that period of service reform some on the Right as well as some in the traditionally Left-wing field of community development argued that the state's role in promoting greater social action is simply to get out of the way. Sometimes the state does indeed get in the way, but what is often needed is a step sideways rather than back. Building on ideas of service 'personalisation' developed by Charlie Leadbeater (Leadbeater, 2004), Geoff Mulgan (Mulgan, 2010; Cooke and Muir, 2012) argued for a 'relational state': government seeing itself not as leader and provider but as convenor and commissioner. The relational state would seek to build relationships with and between people and to work wherever possible through partnerships, communities and networks. Similarly, David Halpern (2010) espouses a 'partner state'.

This book focuses on long-term support to disabled people, older people and other adults and families who may need years or decades of help. Relationships are by definition at the heart of those services and this book attempts to set out ways in which those kinds of public services in particular can find a new relationship with families and communities. This means that professionals would step in earlier but be more reluctant to 'take over'. They would be more realistic about the expertise and capacity that services have and deploy their resources where possible in a supporting role to the capabilities of the people to whom their help was offered, recognising that services on their own often create a poor simulacrum of family and community.

This book argues for a state which is not less resourced, but is scaled down to human size in its approach, enabling us more easily to take on responsibilities which feel shared, safe and manageable. This would both ask more and offer more, and it would be a state which recognises that state money is just one of many resources. It would be more concerned with the risks that matter most to us (loneliness, lacking purpose) and more pragmatic about others.

I started my career working within a care service within an ordinary house and run by an organisation that aspired to provide independence for people with learning disabilities (as well as to make money, in the newly outsourced world of long-term care provision). Subsequently, I worked with unpaid family carers, including children caring for their sick parents, and witnessed their vast, hidden contribution to the welfare state. I also saw how public services were congenitally unable to regard those unpaid carers as their partners, much less their equals, even where untrained, unpaid and unsupported family members were demonstrably achieving more health and happiness for their family member than expensive professional services could even aim for. I now work in the little-known Shared Lives sector, which for decades has quietly been providing long-term support to people with learning disabilities and more recently to a much wider group, in ordinary family homes. If you have a Shared Lives household on your street, you may not even have noticed: you will simply have seen a household in which you can't quite work out how everyone is related.

Shared Lives carers do not fit the accepted description of 'professional': some are registered nurses, but I have met others who are publicans, retired police officers or farmers. Their role is deeply personal and they and their families do much for which they expect no payment, but they are not unpaid volunteers. After an extended approval process, they are matched with adults who need support and it is only when both parties decide they actively want to spend time together that they share home and family life. They are not family carers, but some have lived together as a household for decades and they typically say that the person who lives with them is 'just part of the family'. They talk about fun, laughter and love more than quality or risk management, but this model, which eschews much of the paperwork and process of most public services, is consistently rated as safer and more effective than all those models by government inspectors, while also being demonstrably lower cost.

Crucially, this is a model that has now taken root in almost every area of the UK, supporting nearly 14,000 people and growing while all other care and support sectors are in retreat (Shared Lives Plus, 2017). The experience of working first within the traditional care sector, then supporting unpaid family carers and finally working with people involved in a support model that combines elements of both those worlds, has led me to question almost everything in current public service thinking. It is impossible to witness people's experience of Shared Lives without starting to see traces of the asylum almost everywhere else.

For most policy makers, the asylum is part of public service history. Without clear sight of its malign legacy, attempts to reform public services which offer long-term support have been locked for decades in a cycle of failed initiatives. That failure has become unconscious: simply part of the reality of the public policy world, in which everyone expects government to come up with a plan every couple of years to 'integrate' disjointed services, or to 'shift' resources 'upstream' to prevent crises rather than wait for them, but no one expects those plans to work. This is seen as no one's fault, because no one really believes they have agency over the bureaucracies in which they spend their working lives. Throughout these change and improvement programmes, and their 'task and finish groups', the asylum remains intact and unseen: its assumptions, its relationships, its power dynamics, its iron grasp on scarce resources and its abhorrence of love.

As the first half the book attempts to demonstrate, this is not a 'heritage' issue, in which the outmoded models of the past have been hard to erase. Nor do I believe, as do many working within (or even managing) public services, that we are the subjects and victims of 'the system': a vast, impersonal construct which is impervious to our puny, human attempts at change. There is no abstract system, only us, the relationships between us and the choices we make every day. Currently we choose constantly to ignore, patch up and even rebuild the invisible asylum, whether we are citizens who feel that the council is responsible for our wellbeing and the NHS for our health, or professionals who feel that their expertise is the key to 'fixing' the troublesome patients and customers they are there to 'fix' or 'serve'. Continuing to embed dehumanising practices and the need for building-based services, while wishing to become more 'person focused' and 'community based', crushes those working within our public services just as much as those using them. So the problems that the first chapters of this book identify as fundamental are not those which most commentators consider the most important. In fact, most 'serious' commentators ignore them completely, which is why the new system I outline in the second half has equally little in common with the solutions currently most prominent.

Watching people enjoy their lives in Shared Lives households, receiving support that can be highly sophisticated at times and at others completely improvised, while also contributing more to those around them than many believed possible, has convinced me that we can reject the divide between citizens of our communities and subjects of our services once and for all. We do not have to choose between public services exactly as they stand, or glib reliance on volunteers and the elusive 'big society'. We can combine our own resources and resourcefulness, the love of our families and communities, with the resources, backup and infrastructure of state support.

The second half of this book draws on those public service innovations that have already redesigned themselves around people and their relationships to outline a new model of public services and what its relationships with us could be. These approaches are scattered and small scale, but taken together, they model a completely new system: its ethos, practices, economics and results.

It is far from certain, however, how far into crisis our current system must go before we recognise that the risks of persisting with our current approaches outweigh the risks of radical change. As with climate change, it is also hard to predict what will constitute the point of no return, after which the feedback loops of rising costs, ageing demographics, falling budgets and collapsing consensus lay to waste our much-cherished hospitals and care services. What is certain, however, is that the invisible asylums we have built with such care are overcrowded and crumbling, and that none of us dream of living inside them.

ONE

How we divide the world into community and asylum

When disability happens in your family it is like you wake up in a place you never knew existed, a place that many families refer to as 'service land', where things are often done to you rather than with you. The search for an accurate diagnosis takes over your life, ultimately knowing that if you have a name for what is wrong, this will give you the passport to the support and services that you need. We have created a system which has put people in competition with each other, because our social care system is neither equitable nor transparent, we have made people dependent on the system, by reinforcing that 'the state knows best', yet we have the biggest population across the western world of people with disabilities or support needs who are likely to outlive their family members, this has never happened on such a huge scale before. We have over complicated the lives of people with learning disabilities and their families and need to bring people back to ordinary lives, not just the chosen few living extraordinary lives.

(Caroline Tomlinson, activist, parent and founder of My Life[1])

In the days of workhouses, asylums, debtors' prisons and fever hospitals, it was easy to see who was considered part of their community and who had been removed from the community, for support, punishment or a combination of the two. Most of the most obviously institutional buildings have gone, but the ideas behind that divide between those inside and those outside the community remain invisibly woven into our public services which provide long-term support.

Maintaining that divide can feel comforting, particularly during times in our lives when we do not find ourselves needing state-organised or funded support. Most of us prefer to feel that there is little possibility of state involvement in our lives. People who require long-term support are doubly stigmatised: once through being labelled with the names of stigmatised conditions such as mental ill health, and again, through being seen as having lost capacity, independence, full citizenship. The popular perception of many kinds of support service remains rooted in folk memories of people in uniforms that came to 'take you away' and forbidding Victorian buildings. Ignoring state services is, however, a luxury which few of us can afford to maintain throughout our ever-lengthening lives.

The institutional thinking that remains in our attitudes to public services also means that when we do try to access support within our family homes and our communities, we can find service interventions scarce and under-resourced, as the majority of public service spending is locked in to the remaining buildings such as our increasingly expensive hospitals. Interventions that are organised on a large scale, to cater for hundreds or thousands of people in an area, can feel clumsy and a poor fit with our messy lives and scattered families. Even services that come into our homes usually do so at times arranged around their staff rota, rather than our lives. This is an inevitable part of support organised on a large scale and (despite attempts to 'personalise' services) services are scaling up, rather than down, as the state's care-buyers attempt to reduce unit and transaction costs by having fewer, larger contracts.

At best this is inconvenient, as we have to take time off work or arrange childcare to attend health appointments which are timed and located for the service's efficiency, rather than to fit our lives. But at times in our lives when we need ongoing support, particularly for majority of us who lack the private means to buy it on our own terms, the demands of the services we rely on for

14

support start to eat away at the routines and relationships which keep us connected to family and community life.

The dividing lines between community and the invisible asylum are drawn in a number of ways; this chapter attempts to bring some of them into visibility so that later in the book, we can consider whether they are located in the right places, or indeed, needed at all.

Locking the gates

Relatively few services offered to adults can be accessed freely whenever we feel we need them. The general practitioner (GP) is the totemic example despite relatively long waits in some areas, but it is an exception rather than the rule. GP appointments, usually ten minutes and delivered by increasingly pressured professionals, are themselves increasingly a gatekeeping function for the bulk of NHS services, rather than being a conversation in which an in-depth response or treatment can be offered for all but the most routine illnesses.[2] Nearly every public service intervention starts with a needs assessment. And while many health services remain free, most social care interventions additionally involve a means test, to decide whether people who have been deemed eligible for the service will then be asked to pay for it.

So the needs assessment is the starting point for most public services and it is in the needs assessment that public services start to fail in their missions.

Needs assessments have two, often incompatible, aims: to decide whether the service is useful ('appropriate') for the individual and to ration resources to those most in need. This can often result in a process which feels more a test of whether the individual is appropriate for the service (or is instead an 'inappropriate referral') and where the shared desire of the potential 'service user' and the front-line professional for the individual to get 'in' to the service, is frustrated by the questions and forms they are using, which may well be designed to keep people 'out'.

So, for many, a system which starts with a needs and eligibility assessment, very often also ends there, as the individual is thoroughly and expensively assessed, but then found to be ineligible. As one parent put it to me, "I look at my own son and the amount of energy and effort and cost that's vested in his assessment, then nobody actually follows up until the following year when the amount of money available, inevitably, is checked." Resource-starved people and families and resource-starved front-line practitioners both expend time and money they can ill afford on a fruitless battle with each other.

For example, the Community Care Assessment is the process by which older people and others with long-term or lifelong care and support needs establish their eligibility for adult social care. Progressive changes to social care law have ensured that assessments consider not only what an individual needs and what their problems are, but also what their goals and choices are, and what informal support they receive from family members and others. This is an attempt to create a more rounded picture of the individual's life on which to base their care plan, but, because councils are only legally obliged to support people with substantial enough eligible needs, the experience of a Community Care Assessment remains primarily one in which individuals prove their 'fit' with a service, by virtue of having a high enough level of need. So a sympathetic assessor will advise people to focus not on their capacity but on their 'worst days', which will result in more support being offered. Conversely, identifying the capacity or potential capacity of the individual risks the individual being deemed ineligible. This principle extends to the amount of care offered by a family carer: the more unpaid care the family offers, the less state support the individual gets. As support allocations are increasingly expressed in cash amounts ('personal budgets' are discussed in more detail later), the reduction in those amounts which result from unpaid family care being offered is known, without intended irony, as the 'carers' deflator'.[3]

Assessments are not only a feature of entering a service system; people are also assessed as they attempt to leave it, or to move from a building-based service to a 'community' service. Strangely, given how keen services are to keep people out, in these assessments, they can prove equally anxious to keep the person *in*.

Hospital discharge planning meetings ostensibly aim to avoid 'bed blocking' by speeding the departure of usually elderly patients who are 'medically fit for discharge'. But hospital-based staff can see home as the site of risks which they cannot control, such as the elderly person falling. Conversely, they can struggle to see the risks of the person staying in hospital, such as contracting a hospital 'super bug' like MRSA,[4] or the no less deadly risk of swiftly becoming too frail and dependent to live at home.[5] From a 'professional' point of view, hospital is 'safe'; home is not. Before the health problem or accident that brought the older person into hospital, he or she probably chose to take risks. But once the 'system' has assumed responsibility for the individual, people in responsible roles can feel unable safely to relinquish that responsibility. A colleague asks hospital discharge teams, 'What do we know of this person and what they were capable of a few days ago?' Typically, a room full of experts must admit their collective answer is, 'Nothing'.

In physics, the Observer Effect describes the effect we have on something by observing it. An older person being assessed in a hospital or care home kitchen, to see if they can make a cup of tea (a common test for their readiness to return home after an operation), may well become flustered and disorientated through the stress of being observed. Few of us could parent in a relaxed and confident manner while in a Parenting Assessment Unit, where parents with learning disabilities are assessed, aware that their children are imminently at risk of being removed from their care if they fail.

Needs assessments aim to comprehend the person being assessed, to extract from their collection of traits, experiences, scars and potential, a neat stack of labels, scores and codes, which can be parcelled into the boxes of our public services. Thus, we lose the person in the very process designed to find them.[6] Another idea from physics, Heisenberg's Uncertainty Principle, is that, for certain pairs of properties of particles, such as trajectory and position, the more you knew about one, the less certain you can be of the other. Similarly, the more we can define a person's need, the less we can know of their capacity, whereas if the system gains a clear view of their capacity, their needs can become invisible. So where an individual's health and wellbeing improves, what should be cause for celebration is in fact a moment of great risk: an entitlement that may have been won through battles with assessors that can stretch into years for some groups, can vanish in moments without leaving any trace. Should their progress then falter, the individual may find themselves back at the bottom of the snakes and ladders board, to begin the battle to prove need all over again.

Asylum seekers and revolving doors

People with fluctuating support needs, such as many people with mental health problems or who have a relapsing/remitting health condition like multiple sclerosis, can find the support they need tantalisingly just beyond their reach. When an increase in support needs leads to support being put in place, any success that support has in improving their wellbeing leads to its swift withdrawal. Like the life of a would-be migrant, life just outside the borders of service eligibility can be uncertain and stressful, with days taken up with fruitless form-filling and appointments with assessors. A Shared Lives carer describes how a man with a learning disability had thrived living with her in her supportive household: "So they decide he can manage in supported living, which is just a few hours of support a week. He becomes isolated and can't cope so he ends up in crisis and comes back to us until he's better and they start trying to move him out all over again."

This catch-22 situation is not limited to the health and care system. For example, the social enterprise Community Catalysts supports people with learning disabilities to develop their own 'microenterprises', built on what they can do and learn, as a way in which people can contribute to community life and – potentially – move into paid employment. A young woman with a learning disability who likes bikes and working with food is now part of an enterprise, Pulp Friction, she runs with friends which takes pedal-powered 'smoothie' makers around festivals and events, selling healthy drinks. Any income is currently small and occasional and to use it to pay the disabled workers a wage would be of no financial benefit to them: they would simply have their welfare benefits reduced accordingly. More worrying, by establishing their ability to earn income, they may permanently jeopardise their status as eligible for certain benefits. Their support needs remain considerable and the risk of their enterprising failing or staying extremely small is very high, making it safer all round for the enterprise to remain entirely voluntary and the individuals excluded from the ordinary world of work, which is so strongly associated with full citizenship.

For some, repeatedly being assessed by services that will not support them stems from having multiple support needs. By 2018 it is estimated the number of people with multiple conditions will have grown from 1.9 million to 2.9 million (McShane and Mitchell, 2013). Those nearly 3 million people will be assessed by each condition-specific service or professional, often giving the same information, but with no way for the assessment systems to consider the cumulative impact of multiple conditions, nor to lead to coordinated working between the agencies. Where someone has both medical diagnoses and social challenges, they may be considered 'challenging' or even 'inappropriate' for some services.

For instance, 20%–30% of offenders have learning disabilities and 72% of male and 70% of female sentenced prisoners suffer from two or more mental health disorders. A lack of suitable (or sometimes any) housing has long been identified as key factor in recidivism,[7] but most offenders leave custody with little ongoing housing support (Social Exclusion Unit, 2002). The Revolving Doors agency was set up to tackle the problems faced by people with deep-rooted problems that manifest themselves in self-destructive substance misuse and criminality, leading to them moving constantly between community and medical or criminal justice services. The charity's publicity says: 'Our police, courts and prisons see people in this group every day yet they get little or no effective help from mainstream health and other services.' Each service may spend large amounts on 'supporting' the individual, but each is focused on a single set of needs, none able to see all the needs, let alone the whole person, who will be an individual with goals, capacity and potential. State money, and more importantly, years of people's lives, are wasted.

In contrast to the gatekeeping which polices access to adults' support services, the main children's service, the school, is free and universal. Without the stigma or cost of being rationed or means-tested, schools can be a site in which not only are a wide range of non-educational services offered, from vaccinations to breakfast clubs, but are also places which can fit with and enhance the communities they serve. The parents and grandparents who come in and out of their gates form strong social bonds[8] on which are built activities, committees and a significant chunk of community life. It's notable that this is particularly true of primary schools, which tend to be smaller and more centrally located in a community, as opposed to much larger secondary schools, which must often be reached by car or bus and where fewer parents accompany their children to or inside the school gates.

It is commonly assumed that it is only through increasingly stringent needs assessment that overstretched services are kept from collapse under the weight of unmet need. But, like many assumptions regarded as 'common sense', it has never been tested. What would happen if adult services were made universal? In place of the needs assessment, the gateway intervention could be the creation of a support plan which focus on what the individual and their family can do, or could do with the right help. How many of us would rush headlong for the most expensive, and intrusive, services, if offered lighter touch but effective alternatives?

Being inappropriate

For some time I worked as a care assistant in a residential care home for four men with a learning disability, most of whom had been labelled 'challenging' in some way. The home was staffed mainly by skilled and well-motivated people who wanted to help the men have good lives. There were many positive aspects to the men's lives, particularly in comparison to the large institutions they would have been placed in not that many years previously. The men's behaviour was, in varying ways, not what most people would consider 'appropriate' at various times. Some did not share most people's understanding of appropriate physical contact. Their behaviours could range from being overly tactile to hitting staff members. My main memories of the discussions we had around our interactions with the men revolve around discussions of what was appropriate and how we managed risk. Underlying our ideas of appropriateness was a strong sense of professional boundaries. We were constantly in the role of 'risk assessor', while the men were always in the position of being assessed.

The men spent most of their time with us, paid staff members. They were not in employment so had no colleagues and they had limited social lives, other than occasional social activities with their families or those we took them to. They all found it hard to make and keep friends. Their home was a large and comfortable detached suburban house, but it was also a workplace, with one room acting as an office; staff working shifts (including strangers sent by agencies to fill in for sick staff); staff meetings in the living room and notices on some of the walls. We took it as read that the men should act in a way which was appropriate to their surroundings and relationships, without, to my memory, considering the strange mixture of home and workplace they were living in, or the equally hard-to-define mixture of friend, helper and supervisor we were in our relationships to them. It was seen as vital that our relationships with the men were entirely one-way: the men could not experience us as needing anything from them, so the men had few relationships with anyone who needed anything from them.

If we lived locally and bumped into one of the men when we socialising, we were expected to finish our drink and leave for another venue, in case one of the men saw us intoxicated. Had one of them wished to get drunk themselves, there would have been risk assessments, forms filled in and 'appropriate' boundaries imposed.

It was notable that the men who were occasionally violent, and sometimes physically restrained as a result, were only violent towards staff members. One would appear to lose all self-control during an 'incident', but never, ever struck out at someone in public, or anyone other than a staff member. The staff members had the same rights as anyone else to report violence to the police, but it was accepted that this would never happen and the general view was that if this normal consequence was ever imposed, it would lead to the care arrangement breaking down and some sort of more institutional care. I often wonder now what would have happened if the normal rules of community, which existed in the street outside and the houses next door, had been applied within 'the service'. Staff, residents and relatives all shared a belief that this was unthinkable.

What was appropriate to such an unusual environment? We expected the men to navigate their relationships with us with a skill that would have eluded most people, let alone someone with a learning disability, additional mental health problems and in some cases long spells in institutions. We were wary of being manipulated by shows of affection. We discussed often how to 'de-escalate' the men's 'challenging behaviour' but it did not occur to me that challenging the environment we had created might in fact be entirely 'appropriate', nor that expressing anger 'inappropriately' was normal behaviour for all of us at times.

It is impossible to say now to what extent the men's behaviour was facilitated or exacerbated by our expectation of 'appropriate' behaviour, within an environment and within relationships which would not be experienced by most of us as remotely ordinary or OK. However, it is striking that, even in this 'community setting', some of the aspects of life which most of us take for granted as fundamental to living well – living among our chosen friends or our families, taking risks, making mistakes, getting angry, suffering consequences – were altered or absent in these men's lives, despite the warmth, dedication and skills of the people I met on my shifts.

My experience of working as a care assistant was some years ago, but the sector's belief in professional boundaries and appropriate behaviour persists. In adult care and support, it is perhaps only the Shared Lives model which allows participants to talk of 'love', without triggering a safeguarding investigation.

When the people working in services come under stress, particularly in an environment of chronic under-resourcing and ever-increasing pressure, adherence to professional boundaries can warp our humanity completely out of shape.

In 2014, Sally M., 22, took two overdoses, having spent years with a serious eating disorder and personality disorder and having a long history of self-harming. She was seen by her community psychiatric team and crisis staff from a NHS Foundation Trust, where several members of staff recommended admission to hospital. On Friday 25 July, Sally pleaded to be taken into a unit, saying she was going to kill herself. Allegedly two mental health nurses in the crisis team sent her home after a 14-minute assessment, using four staff to restrain her, then calling the police to have her removed when she started banging her head on a wall and tried to strangle herself in her distress. The police officers were so concerned at her distress that they tried to change the nurses' minds, unsuccessfully. She killed herself two hours later. The coroner ruled that Sally's death was a direct result of the failure to admit her to the unit and said the NHS Trust caused "unimaginable and unnecessary suffering", for which the incoming Chief Executive of the Trust apologised on the last day of the inquest, and more than a year after the event.

This incident is an aberration which will appal most mental health professionals but, while their conduct was heavily criticised, the nurses defended their behaviour in the inquest, stating that they felt that her behaviour that day was part of a 'chronic' rather than 'acute' pattern and therefore not a sign that she had become significantly more likely to kill herself, which would justify an admission. They appear to have become inured to extreme behaviour and deeply cynical about it. That cynicism seems extreme, but I can see it reflected in cynicism and dark humour I have heard from others who have spent years working with people with similar conditions and who know what it is like to feel 'burnt out'.

For every public scandal, there are countless thousands of unnoticed Friday afternoons in which equally weary, undervalued and under-resourced health workers are faced with a 'difficult' person with a long history of self-destructive or manipulative behaviour, and who make the best choices they can with compassion.

One of the nurses was reported by the police officers as saying of her use of a ligature, "Leave her to faint. She will faint before she dies. We can take it off her then". The police officers, perhaps less immersed in the mental health system, begged for a hospital admission and even encouraged the staff to make a complaint against Sally so that they could arrest her and take her to a police cell, as a safer place than home. Eventually, they reluctantly took her home, feeling powerless to do otherwise. In this instance, the nurses allegedly behaved with a by-the-book lack of empathy which people might expect of hardened police officers, while the police empathised with the suffering and felt powerless to intervene.[9]

While most people working in public services do so with inspiring reserves of compassion and skill, it is not surprising that many who work for long periods at the point of interaction between dehumanising system and unwell or desperate humans will start to despair. Some will be themselves so deeply damaged by that despair, they will start to personify the unfeeling, amoral systems within which they work.

I've often heard mental health professionals say their first goal in working with a new patient is keeping them out of the mental health system. What does that say about that system and the people who work in it? First it says that those mental health professionals care. They do not ignore and are not complacent about the negative impacts of services. It also says that professionals see what they do – caring for others – as distinct from 'the mental health system'. I've never heard one say, 'the important thing is to ensure that this person has as little contact with *me* as possible'. We don't see our own, individual interventions as being damaging; it's 'the system' which is damaging. So what is 'the system'? To many, it is the product of institutional processes, pathways, economics, buildings and stigma. The system is, I believe, also the choices and relationships which all of us who live or work within it make – and feel we cannot make – every day.

So the nature of the system cannot be separated from the profile of the people working within it and their relative share of power. Our current health and care systems become more male-dominated and less ethnically diverse the further up the chain of command you go. So what the system sees as 'appropriate' will in many cases derive from a white, male, Western view of culture, relationships and communication styles, and the actions of people from for instance, BME (black and minority ethnic) communities using a service will be interpreted through the assumptions of those in power, or the limitations of their ability to listen to and communicate with people from different communities to their own.

The very act of providing and receiving care within a bureaucracy can widen between the role prescribed for care professionals and their caring emotions. It is narrowed when people have no choice but to relate more personally to each other (for instance, when people who taken Direct Payments directly employ a small team of staff, as explored in Chapter Five), but also when people have the courage to reject it, resisting the power structures within which they meet each other.

The problem with being a customer

It is worth paying attention to the words systems use; they can reveal underlying beliefs. When medics talk about 'my patient', who may be 'under' a certain physician or hospital, they say something about their working relationships and power. Medical bodies whose boards or committees have members who lack medical qualifications refer to them as 'lay' members: thus medics ordain themselves as a priesthood. Changing the language used within organisations and systems can often be a substitute for changing behaviour and beliefs, with the new softer-sounding language adding a coating of irony to unyielding bureaucracies.

One of the ways in which many public services have tried to indicate a change of relationship with the people they support is through the widespread practice of referring to people as 'customers'. Many councils describe the people who live in their local area not as citizens, but as customers. They operate 'customer service' centres. Importing customer service culture from the private sector service industries was one way in which the Blair government attempted to 'modernise' services which had previously called people 'service users'.

Being a 'customer' (or 'client' in some services) sounds better than being a 'service user', but it is worth thinking about exactly what that status implies. Customers buy their way into a contract with an organisation that wants their money. But most of us approach public services either with no money, because the service does not charge, or having proved our relative poverty to pass a means test. People choosing care and support services, like care homes, often do so in a crisis, encountering a limited range of confusing choices, none of which may feel like they match the life they imagined themselves living. These 'customers' find they have little power even when spending a great deal of their own money, but those customers who are spending very limited amounts of the state's money, have fewer choices and less power. They may be called customers, but feel like supplicants.

Setting aside the power dynamics at play, when we choose or buy long-term support, we are seeking not just a service, but a relationship with the person or people who will provide that support. Ultimately, we cannot be customers of relationships.

A customer is someone who has some rights, but few responsibilities. As a customer of a shop I do not control what the shop sells. If it is a local corner shop I may be friendly with the owner and able to make suggestions, but not if it is a large supermarket. I will argue shortly that there are some fundamental design flaws in our long-term support services, which will only be fixed when those services are co-designed with the people who use them. Customers not only lack the power to design anything; it is not their responsibility to do so.

A person's interaction with any support service will be most cost-effective where both service and individual (or family) bring their energy, time and creativity and where they see success as a shared responsibility, not something which one party owes the other. This only happens where the workers and people can form real relationship. It is better to be a citizen than a customer.

Professionals and amateurs

Public services operate hierarchies within their teams, based on the level of qualification of practitioners, or the size of budget controlled by managers. People with long-term conditions who remain living in their own homes usually receive most of the care they need from their partner or relatives, but neither the hours of care provided nor the expertise they develop in doing so qualifies unpaid family carers to even the bottom rung of those hierarchies, despite the unpaid care provided by families and friends worth well over £100 billion and rising: comparable to the combined values of formal health and social care (both of which are shrinking).

Family carers have campaigned for and achieved important rights, but a comparison of their entitlements and those which any paid care or health worker would expect, illustrates that carers are recognised as a group of people with support needs, but not as equal partners of public service professionals. So the key right is to a separate needs assessment. Some of those who care 24/7 have limited rights to a break. There is no right to a sustainable household income, beyond the entitlement for some to a welfare benefit of £62.70 per week (2017/18 rate). A paid worker taking on an all-consuming caring role for someone with complex medical needs expects induction, training, essential equipment, relevant information, access to experts when needed and emergency backup during a crisis. A family carer can expect none of these. Indeed, there is a well-developed literature, which frames families as a common part of the problem. While unevidenced theories about 'schizogenic' and 'refrigerator' mothers (blamed for their offspring's mental illnesses or autism, respectively) are long-since discredited, it is still common to hear talk of 'over-protective' parents of people with learning disabilities, which can sometimes be justified, but can also conveniently overlook a family's repeated experiences of being excluded or let down by services whose promises did not outlast a policy, budget or staffing change, leaving the family to pick up the pieces.

The different value placed on family care is not indicative of its real value nor its complexity. In June 2011, the BBC's investigative programme, *Panorama*, exposed appalling abuse at an 'Assessment and Treatment Centre' called Winterbourne View. The centre was a facility ostensibly for the assessment and treatment of people with learning disabilities whose additional mental health needs and 'challenging behaviour' were classed as health, rather than social care needs, thus making their care wholly or jointly an NHS responsibility. Many of the residents, whose needs were considered so complex that they needed medical care costing up to £5,000 per week each, had lived with their families into early adulthood. Their families generally had no training, few if any breaks from caring, no backup from services when there was a crisis and none of the status or respect of (even unqualified) professionals. Some will have been in difficult financial circumstances due to one or both parents caring rather than being in paid work and the additional costs of disability in the family such as the costs of equipment or adaptations not available on the NHS. Similarly, many older people receive intensive support from poorly supported partners or family members desperate to delay the admission to a care home they know will not be reversed.

When family care arrangements break down, care assessments and support professionals often have lots to say about the ways in which unpaid carers have 'failed' to manage behaviour, provide 'appropriate' boundaries, and 'support independence'. The same professionals will describe the failures of their own interventions much more forgivingly: it is the individual's 'lack of progress', not the service's; the 'treatment' was 'indicated', but the individual has 'not responded' or was 'non-compliant'.

That untrained, unpaid and unsupported family carers could help their relative to live a 'good enough' life, while highly resourced, regulated and 'professional' services could not, suggests we are missing something. Perhaps there are design flaws in our long-term support services which run too deep for us to see, just as there appear to be equally profound strengths and capacity within some families, which are invisible to services. If paid support is often a very poor and expensive substitute for the care and love found within most families, that is a flaw unlikely to be fixed by more regulations, training, inspections or even money. To try to do so could just be to continue to direct resources to precisely the wrong place (building-based services) or precisely the wrong time (just after family life breaks down).

This is not to say that everyone with support needs could or should be cared for by their families. Not all family members are willing and able to provide ongoing substantial care to their relative. Not everyone wants to receive intimate care from relatives, or to let their families take decisions for them; for instance, most young disabled adults dream of a place of their own. To attempt to force either party into an unpaid caring situation would be disastrous for both.

But to give and receive long-term care within a family is a valid choice. At present, it can be a choice that risks the family's emotional and financial sustainability, while relinquishing any claim on the resources available to the state.

What would happen to our experiences, and to the economics of our public services, if it was possible to make a more balanced choice between family and service-based care? If families could access the same resources, training, backup and respect which 'professionals' expect? And people working in services could form relationships which felt more real and human? We might view the relative risks and capabilities of families and staff teams quite differently, and combine the state's limited resources with families' limited resources through service approaches that tried to draw the best from both worlds.

"Don't call me a service user, I'm a professional just like you"

CHANGE, a disabled-people-led organisation based in Leeds, is rare in the sector in using a 'co-worker' model, in which it employs someone with a learning disability alongside a non-disabled post-holder, on equal salaries, terms and conditions. Shaun Webster MBE, a trainer and European Co-ordinator with CHANGE, describes how he had worked previously in a warehouse where he felt of little value and was bullied. In contrast, he now speaks at conferences in the UK and Europe and is regarded as an expert. He particularly values the fact that where there are other people with learning disabilities, sometimes including children, in the audience, he can be a role model and inspiration for them. Shaun gets extremely frustrated by the common practice in the UK of holding conferences about learning disability in which only one person with a learning disability is engaged as a speaker, still less anyone in a paid role. At one conference, Shaun and his colleagues all ended their presentations by saying, "Don't call me a service user. I'm a professional just like you". CHANGE refuses to separate the question of how to improve care for people with the highest support needs from the deeper structural and cultural oppression that those people experience through lacking basic rights to housing, freedom from discrimination, a voice and paid employment. In 2014/15 48% of disabled men and 44% of disabled women were in employment compared to 84 % and 74% of non-disabled men and women (MacInnes et al, 2015). This large gap is falling slowly, but the proportion of learning disabled people in work is only 6% and falling (Learning Disabilities Observatory, 2016).

Clearly, there are many roles that are likely to prove challenging for people with an intellectual or developmental impairment, but it is striking that many roles that could and arguably should be filled by people with intellectual and other impairments are not. Even some organisations whose purpose is to support people with learning disabilities into paid employment, and who receive government funding to do so, do not appear to employ disabled people in paid leadership roles. The usual approach within the learning disability sector is to attempt to support people into menial roles or to create courses to help them become 'work ready'. Work or skills-oriented day activities appear more 'inclusive' and aspirational than the day centres and 'sheltered' workplaces they replaced, in which people worked for years on repetitive menial tasks for token amounts of money, but many people spend years in 'preparation' for opportunities which never materialise.

But there are existing well-paid roles in which lived experience of having a learning disability could be recognised as an advantage, particularly if a co-worker model was adopted. For instance, the Care Quality Commission (CQC) has found that service inspectors who have a learning disability can be good at recognising good and poor care, as well as challenging workers' assumptions about the status of disabled and non-disabled people as colleagues. They may have more potential to connect with other people with learning disabilities and empathise with their experiences. (These 'experts by experience' roles were outsourced by CQC, however, and pay reduced to the National Living Wage.) CHANGE and other user-led organisations have found that mixed-ability teams can be more effective at training workers or delivering health education and some kinds of advocacy.

So, the choice of people for paid roles within public services is important to the impact of that work, but it is also a rarely examined expression of the power divides embedded within those services. Even large campaigning charities, whose business is empowerment, have in many cases not addressed the power balances within their own structures, which divide people into those who need support and those who provide it.

The parallels with the civil rights and gender equalities movements are clear, but never discussed by policy makers, because older people in the adult support system are beyond retirement age and it is assumed that working-age adults are less employable. However, equality for oppressed and marginalised groups never comes from appealing to the better nature of the groups who hold the power, but only from members of the affected group themselves gaining powerful positions.

Escaping the invisible asylum: actions

1. See all of the person not just all of the needs

Every front-line public services worker and manager will find themselves in situations where an individual's life, circumstances and needs are under intense scrutiny. Focusing only on identifying their needs may result in 'losing the person'. This will be a particular risk where the group assessing people lacks the diversity of the community it assesses. The presenting moment contains evidence only of an individual's crisis: their risks, needs and pathology. These form a scant set of tools to work with. Learn who the person was before they met you and who they wish to be when they leave you.

2. Relearn humility

Looking for capabilities and potential of people and their families requires a humility that is trained or conditioned out of many professions, particularly those that employ few people with lived experience. Relearning that humility will also bring with it the confidence of having a clear view of what we can and cannot do. This is healthier than the guilt of the professional who feels trapped in an inhuman system, or the brittle status anxiety of the 'expert'.

3. Support the emotionally and financially sustainable household

The creation of emotionally and financially sustainable households needs to become a key policy priority. Households need to be able to plan together as well as separately and to pursue employment alongside caring responsibilities. This requires services willing to fit within the individual's support ecosystem.

TWO

How we create problems by trying to fix them

> Some people say that community starts in mystery
> and ends in bureaucracy. They start with great
> enthusiasm and a love that surpasses all frontiers, and
> end up with a lot of administration and wealth, loss
> of enthusiasm and fear of risk.
> (Vanier, 1979: 108)

Vanier's description of unintended consequences suggests mystery in the impetus to build collectively, and bafflement at the dysfunctional results. In a similar vein, Ivan Illich took the concept of iatrogenesis, the illness inadvertently caused by the intervention of a doctor, and applied it to public services (Illich, 1974); an idea developed by John McKnight (1995), who used the metaphor of the mechanised John Deere plough turning land, fertile when farmed less intensively by Native Americans, into a dust bowl. So, for McKnight, the overdevelopment of the profession of bereavement counsellor fosters the idea that grief is unhealthy and unmanageable by non-professionals. Grief, which was previously a 'common property' of the community – a shared responsibility to which family, friends and neighbours would respond – has become the exclusive professional domain of experts who are licensed and funded to assist the individual to process it:

> Like John Deere's plow, the tools of bereavement
> counseling will create a desert where a community
> once flourished.

33

> And finally, even the bereavement counselor will
> see the impossibility of restoring hope in clients once
> they are genuinely alone, with nothing but a service
> for consolation. In the inevitable failure of the service,
> the bereavement counselor will find the desert even
> in herself. (McKnight, 1995: 7)

By extension, any public service that operates in an area of life
that was previously the domain of ordinary family or community
relationships risks 'colonising' that area of life, creating 'careless
societies' with clients rather than citizens, who lack confidence
in their ability to care for themselves and each other.

McKnight's ideas have not taken hold among UK service
planners or policy makers. They are deeply uncomfortable for
those who do not wish to think of themselves as doing more
harm than good with the resources they control, but also for
activists and people who rely on services for vital support and
feel those services are increasingly attacked and cut.

Taken to their logical conclusion, McKnight's argument
could be reduced to an extreme 'small-state' position: cut
as many services as possible to get them out of the way of
people's self-reliance. Some advocates of Prime Minister David
Cameron's 'Big Society', whose slogan was 'Big Society, not
Big Government', appeared to believe social action is always
spontaneous and citizen-led, while state action is always
bureaucratic and infantilising. But, while such community
action starts as a reaction to a gap or reduction in services
(often springing from protests against those very cuts), there is
no evidence to suggest that this community action can replace,
let alone exceed the impact of, public services. Despite this
period of austerity's rapid and sweeping reductions in the size
of the state, the spontaneous flowering of 'community' remains
wishful thinking.

Community action tends to be most effective in building the
kinds of low-level support (befriending, advising) and informal
activities (clubs, gatherings) that benefit people who are not
at great risk, nor in crisis. Community building can reduce
the risk that stress placed on people or households becomes
a full-blown crisis, but a community's cohesion and resilience

cannot eliminate those risks, particularly for those least able to engage with others or most likely to be excluded from or even oppressed by that community. Little community action is entirely unsupported by the state, which provides small grants and use of buildings. During austerity, 'non-essential' community groups and facilities like libraries have often been first to be cut.

Few of us would prefer to rely on an unpaid volunteer than a trained and accountable professional, for personal care or medicine, or when our lives are falling apart on multiple fronts. The professional intervention of a bereavement counsellor may indeed be the best remedy for grief which has remained 'stuck' for many years.

Iatrogenesis is a useful concept in challenging the mindless application of traditional service-thinking (bring in experts to fix these poor people's problems) to every social challenge, but it needs tempering. Vanier founded L'Arche movement in which disabled and non-disabled people live communally. He identified in *Community and Growth* that the main challenge to a growing community is 'to adapt its structures so that they go on enabling the growth of individuals and do not merely conserve a tradition, still less a form of authority and prestige' (Vanier, 1979: 108). The same is true of developing a long-term support model, if we want that model to feel more like community and less like bureaucracy. That challenge cannot be avoided, however pure our intentions. Even the Asset-Based Community Development Institute, which McKnight co-founded and which breathes life into community organising around the world, is also an Institute, whose people accumulate tradable expertise as they dip in and out of communities on their global travels. But equally, a bureaucracy is just a community of people that has progressed too far down the road Vanier predicts; that group of people can choose the difficult, narrowing path back again. Later I outline a public service model that recognises some level of iatrogenesis as inevitable, developing self-awareness to bring negative side effects into visibility, rather than believing any model can be 'perfect'.

In today's cuts-hit public services, 'over-provision' could be seen as a rapidly decreasing risk: most of us would have to wait months or years for a state-funded bereavement counsellor. However, while services are retrenching, belief in their necessity and efficacy is not and the most medicalised and 'formal' interventions remain at the top of the public service pyramid: the last to go as the pyramid sinks into the sand. So people can find they can access no support provision before a crisis, then over-provision of one of the most intrusive forms of support: the 'all or nothing' nature of our support systems is exacerbated by cuts.

Large-scale services for human-scale problems

Service systems, designed to interact with large populations in 'safe' standardised ways, can feel misaligned with the close, personal, reciprocal and risky nature of ordinary human relationships. While the visible depersonalisation inherent in asylum wards and inmates' uniforms may be largely in the past, public services are still inhabited by attempts to offer uniform services to individuals with very different needs, goals and capabilities.

For instance, many agencies delivering home care to older people have large teams and an economic model based on scheduling brief visits around the most efficient journey for the available employees. They employ largely unqualified staff, recruited through a brief process and paid minimum wage.

The BBC reported in May 2012[1] that a woman recorded 106 different workers were sent to care for her husband, whose dementia made consistent relationships vital. A UK Home Care Association survey found that 73% of home-care visits in England were 30 minutes or shorter. 10% of visits lasted just 15 minutes: barely time to help a frail, older person get up washed, dressed and fed (UKHCA, 2012). Providers accepted that this put people's dignity at risk. An Equality and Human Rights Commission inquiry into the home-care system in England found evidence of poor treatment of older people which 'amounts to human rights breaches' and often goes 'undiscovered and unresolved' (EHRC, 2011: 5, 9). A parliamentary committee found that nearly a quarter of care workers administer medication they are not trained for (CLG, 2017).

A 2012 BBC investigation[2] revealed that 200 home-care providers in England had been using staff who had not been properly checked for suitability; people with criminal records were working unsupervised in older people's homes. A 2017 BBC investigation revealed over 23,000 allegations of abuse against home-care workers supporting older and disabled people, including 3,500 allegations of physical abuse and 400 of sexual abuse.[3]

As councils have become more financially desperate during austerity, they are trying to reduce their unit and transaction costs through having fewer, larger contracts, in ways likely to exacerbate the problems. 'Reverse auctions' give care contracts to the cheapest bidder while eligibility thresholds are raised and care packages, supposedly based on individual needs assessments, cut across the board. This results not only in the human cost of poor care and too frequent failure and abuse, but hidden financial costs: to families who have to spend savings or leave employment to care, and in the costs of exceptionally high staff turnover: half of care workers leave within a year of starting (CLG, 2017). A writer in *The Guardian* gave a bleak account of a home-care role:

> I was handed a zero-hours contract to sign and told that I would be paid the national minimum wage of £7.20 an hour…
>
> After just four days of basic training I was sent out to work alongside another care worker. The work itself involved everything from changing incontinence pads and stoma bags to administering medicines and cleaning up some fairly stomach-churning mess. I would usually meet a colleague at around 7 am or 8 am; we would visit service users for 30-minute windows until around 2 pm when we would break for lunch; we would then go back on duty at 4 pm and we would finish at around 10.30 pm. (Bloodworth, 2017)

Even where the support is of 'high quality' in terms of the practical tasks it aims to carry out, there is little time for social support, so 'pervasive social isolation and loneliness [is] experienced by many older people confined to their homes who lack support to get out and take part in community life' (EHRC, 2011: 4). Loneliness in old age is not just miserable, it is also associated with falls, poor physical and mental health and higher risks of dying prematurely, all of which creates further costs in the acute parts of the system, which suck in an ever-increasing share of the available resources.

There is a strong case for many medical procedures being carried out on a large scale in big buildings, which can become centres for technical expertise and getting the most use out of expensive equipment. But where the most important factor in success is the relationship between worker and individual, a large standing team of staff, or a building with beds which must be filled to keep a service viable, become barriers rather than assets. A Healthwatch England inquiry into home care found that some people 'felt that care packages were designed to meet the needs of the service provider rather than the service user' (Healthwatch England, 2017: 10). Smaller home-care providers and smaller care homes are both associated with higher inspection ratings according to CQC, but both are closing or leaving the state-funded market at a higher rate than their larger counterparts, driving an increase in the average size of care providers, away from the small and homely models people seem most to enjoy (CQC, 2017).

Where the staff of large organisations are kind and caring, this success is interpreted as stemming from strong 'organisational culture'. Organisational culture is often described in terms which suggest it is slightly mysterious. A typical definition is the 'system of shared assumptions, values and beliefs, which governs how people behave in organisations'. How do people come to share those assumptions, values and beliefs? Manuals stress the importance of leadership: a strong culture emerges when messages from the top are about compassion, dignity and quality and leaders are seen to model that behaviour. Most large organisations have ways to celebrate front-line workers who rise above the confines of their roles and 'go the extra mile'; they are held up as examples to which everyone should aspire. Meanwhile, those organisations' HR teams deal with a steady stream of performance issues, stress-related sickness and safeguarding concerns.

To senior managers, variations in quality and safety can seem like the inevitable messiness of employing and supporting large numbers of humans. In reality, the proportion of good and poor staff behaviour does not arise just from intangible 'culture'; it is a product of very tangible recruitment, reward and blame systems. In large care organisations, those systems typically start with brief recruitment processes followed by low pay, a focus on carrying out tasks quickly, rigidly prescribed roles and blame-heavy responses to deviance from the norm. Health and care organisations are full of senior leaders who talk eloquently about compassion and dignity, and middle managers whose performance is almost entirely measured against the volume, speed and unit cost of caring tasks their teams achieve. Front-line staff live with the pressures passed down through junior managers, while enduring the inspirational words of senior managers. The rewards for conspicuous compassion may be a glowing staff bulletin article, but the consequences of struggling to maintain a frenetic pace of 'caring' or a maximum case load, are likely to be severe.

While senior managers are expected to articulate a positive vision and culture, they are fundamentally held accountable for their organisation's balance sheet above all else. NHS Trusts which are perpetually in the red lose their chief executives. However, as several high-profile scandals have illustrated, it is much rarer for a CEO to lose their job over failings of compassion or even safety and common to hear a leader talk about their 'responsibility' to stay on, to make the very changes they have failed to understand or prioritise previously.

Southern Health NHS Trust eventually admitted liability for the negligent death of Connor Sparrowhawk. In the investigations that followed, Southern Health was found to have failed to investigate hundreds of unexplained deaths of people with learning disabilities and mental health problems. Its chief executive, a winner of *Health Service Journal* Chief Executive of the Year with a reputation for successful leadership of large change programmes, refused to resign for three years, before a new Chair eventually moved her to a custom-made strategic advisor role on the same salary, followed by a quiet departure (Siddique, 2016). It was another year before the entire board resigned following a damning inspectors' report.

Mid Staffordshire Hospital became notorious after numerous deaths of older people and extensive failings detailed in the lengthy Francis Report. It is difficult to say how many 'extra' deaths had been caused by poor care (you expect lots of people to die from their health conditions in any hospital), but the higher estimates were over a thousand. The report found that the organisation had become focused on the financial requirements of becoming an independent NHS Foundation Trust, which the government and sector saw as the key marker of success in a well-run NHS hospital; in short: balancing the books at any cost. Applying for Foundation Trust status was 'driven by the focus of the process as a whole on financial and corporate governance and not clinical standards' (Francis, 2013, Executive Summary: 50).

Perhaps it says something about our collective view of the value of older people's lives that, while individual nurses were struck off, there were so few consequences for senior managers in the Trust and the region's oversight bodies. Many went on to have national careers, such as Sir David Nicholson who ran England's entire NHS.[4]

People do not forge successful senior careers through maintaining a small-scale, human focus, but through meeting the hard financial challenges of large-scale operations. The more they can align themselves to the macro-scale world, the more power, in the form of large budgets and teams, they wield. And the less well-placed they will be to witness, challenge and change the financial pressures gripping the relationships between front-line workers and people they support. The macro-scale will also be a poor position from which to understand the diversity of the communities they support, particularly as groups of senior managers tend to lack diversity.

It will only be when we require all health and care services to identify and focus on the goals which feel most important to us as humans, which are also the source of sustainable wellbeing (such as feeling in control of one's life or staying connected to others) that the medical and economic logic of operating on a human scale will become inescapable. As discussed in Chapters Seven and Eight, when we devolve money and decision-making power to individuals and small groups, they can behave very differently from the people contained by large organisations, providing the whole system is aligned around (paid for and inspected on) a small set of human goals.

But the larger our services grow, the more resources they pull in from our cash-starved public service economies. They require the most complex and resource-intensive commissioning, planning and management to cope with the huge harm they can cause if they fail. Their managers are the best paid and most powerful. They attract the most expensive research projects. Thus they pull in money, power and talent until they collapse in on themselves and become the black holes of the public service world.

How preventative interventions create crises

'Prevention', along with 'integration' and 'innovation' is one of the most used and abused terms within public service reform. 'Prevention is better than cure' is common sense, but it is very obvious that most money is spent on services that attempt to fix people up after a crisis, with relatively little spent on 'early interventions' that aim to prevent crises. So NHS planners, for instance, talk relentlessly about the need to move health resources from the acute to the community sector. In the jargon, this is pushing resources 'upstream'. It is so self-evidently the right thing to do, that the universal inability to make any progress towards achieving it is discussed as if it were an inconvenient law of nature, like the terrible British weather, which is disappointing but cannot be anyone's fault. Given the deluge of need for crisis services, trying to push resources upstream takes on a Canute-like futility and it starts to seem better to accept the public service world's unfortunate natural laws and go with the flow, rather than look foolish.

One of the problems with prevention is that the concept sounds simple but is interpreted in multiple and often fuzzy ways. The work of the group looking at prevention and early intervention as part of drafting the 2012 Social Care White Paper[5] found that the term 'prevention' was confusing and hard to pin down (successful prevention means something bad did *not* happen, but how can you know that something would have happened but has not?).

It was also seen as negatively formulated and medicalising. As one disability rights activist who has a lifelong condition said, "It sounds like you are dividing disabled people up into two groups of problems: those who can be prevented and those, like me, who can't."

'Prevention' is often used interchangeably with 'early intervention', which describes attempts to reach groups who are at risk, with 'light touch' interventions before they reach crisis point. Investment in doing this seeks only to shift, not remove, the boundary between community life and life within the invisible asylum. While acute and crisis services are legally defined, mandated and regulated, and take up the lion's share of public service budgets, preventative or early interventions are optional, low cost and often rely heavily on volunteers. Individuals have legal rights to acute services once they breach statutory thresholds of need or illness; below those thresholds, they have no individual right to a preventative service (*The Care Act 2014* obliges every English council to have at least some preventative services for disabled adults and older people but this duty is hard to enforce). The care taken with designing early interventions reflects their lower costs, risks and status; many are funded on and through short-term grants to the voluntary sector. Their activities and impacts are not routinely measured, so evidence for them being good uses of public money remains weak. There are no big jobs or power bases within preventative services, towards which ambitious managers or local politicians might gravitate.

An expert on the use of social care resources, Professor John Bolton, writes:

> In the last decade, evidence has further emerged that a little bit of help may be bad for the person. When a person stops carrying out tasks that they could previously undertake with some difficulty they are likely to experience some deterioration in their condition. One of the studies ... even suggests that this can speed the pathway to the need for

further services and increases the likelihood of death. Therefore, the new evidence suggests that what was previously described as preventive actions may in fact offer the opposite for some people... [T]hose councils with the more generous (higher thresholds) of eligibility also had the highest admissions to residential care. (Bolton, 2016: 14)

In contrast to the perverse consequences of some 'preventative' interventions, London School of Economics research found genuinely preventative aspects to time banking, which helps people to contribute as well as receive support (typically through trading an hour of their own time volunteering for an hour of support from someone else) and to befriending, which recognises the value of relationships in supporting good mental health and resilience (Knapp et al, 2011). These interventions take an 'asset-based' approach: they help people to build their own strengths, capabilities and resilience, and those of their families and friends. Later, I will argue that replacing talk of 'prevention' and 'early intervention' with a focus on building and maintaining capacity and resilience, no matter the person's level of need, would give us a genuine chance of success from both a human and a service perspective.

Escaping the invisible asylum: actions

1. The future is small and personal

Government is constantly faced with vast challenges, so understandably tends to favour big solutions. Unfortunately, they nearly always become bureaucracies and institutions. Government should devolve responsibility and resource control to the most personal level possible, then create ways for individuals, households and communities to pool those resources and build towards a scale which works for them. The future of public services will be organised by smartphone, not manufactured on a production line.

2. Stop accepting that we do the wrong things and do the right ones

Who decreed that we should continue to do the things we know do not work, forever? The risks of the status quo, which teeters on the edge of collapse, make the risks of change look positively attractive in comparison. If we accept that new approaches will by their nature lack evidence, let's stop waiting for that evidence and start scaling up whatever has some prospect of working better. Prevention rarely works, but building resilience is always the right outcome and connecting to others is the greatest part of resilience.

3. Aggregating resources builds in inequality

Where health and care resources are managed at a very large scale, by predominantly white managers looking for simplicity, minority groups will be least well served. This is an argument for both scaling down the approach, and for increasing diversity within management teams.

THREE

Why failure pays, but success costs

Jen had left school and we were negotiating with adult's services for the first time. Life beyond school challenged the local council who had one fixed viewpoint: to save money in the short term, achieving survival and ticks in boxes without any consideration of long-term negative consequences. Jen has Down's Syndrome but also a career goal. Jen's dream has remained constant. She wants to share her passion for dance and get the world dancing. We had worked out a plan for her to house-share with a dancer friend via the Shared Lives route and Jen would continue her dance classes. The council's learning disability team leader barely listened when we went to meet him. He said our plan was very interesting but what Jen would actually get was a supported flat, five hours of support a week and a place at the local college. Presumably he already had those contracts in place and the money tied up in them, regardless of what Jen's dreams were.

(Sue Blackwell, co-founder with Jen Blackwell of DanceSyndrome Community Interest Company)

The price of everything, the value of nothing

I suggested in the preceding chapter that the economics of service provision systems are incapable of financially rewarding prevention or recovery, despite these being the outcomes on which everyone in the system agrees as most desirable. Commissioners pay only for the maintenance of high levels of support and crisis. Why?

Public services are set up around specific areas of need: health, social support needs, housing, offender management, substance misuse. Where these are broad, services departmentalise. If you have multiple health conditions, as nearly 3 million of us will have by 2018 (Department of Health, 2012), you will be 'under' different hospital departments for each, with perhaps only your GP in a position to see them all and consider their interrelationship with each other and with you as a person, but too hard-pressed to do so in your ten-minute appointment.

Each part of the system focuses on the part of you that it is there to fix, and having fixed it, or failed to fix it, moves you on as swiftly as possible. The part of the system which sounds like it should be the most holistic, social care, is in fact, for adults, mainly there to provide functional support: brief home visits and price-squeezed care homes with budgets set around minimum wage levels. There are exceptions to this of course: older people's care homes rated outstanding by inspectors which manage to build an atmosphere of warmth and fun from their shoestring budgets, but many of the highest performing home-care and care-home services are privately funded by families wealthy enough to pay for their own care, and thus closed to those relying state funding. Even these typically aim to 'look after' people well, not to enable the person to look after themselves.

It is worth noting here that health, care and other public services are now based around the purchaser/provider split. This means that control of services is devolved to local areas, with one group of organisations in charge of purchasing the service and another group delivering it. In healthcare, both organisations are typically local NHS bodies, with relatively limited numbers of private-sector providers. In social care and housing, the council is the commissioner while most providers have been independent (mainly private sector, but also charities) for years. The theory behind this split is that commissioners will be able to choose between providers, who will compete on price and quality, resulting in innovation and better value for money. The system rests on the skill of commissioners in using their purchasing power to enable, cajole and resource providers to innovate and improve, but many commissioners lack these skills and, during austerity, increasingly they lack the buying power too. Many come from financial backgrounds and have no experience of working in the services they commission. Their 'commissioning' is in reality procurement: buying stuff, as cheaply as possible.

(Some areas have even outsourced their buying power to privately run procurement services run by such unlikely public service experts as BT, the telecoms firm. It is a fundamental duty of public bodies to build and maintain public services. If they neither deliver nor commission those services, what are those bodies for? In the early 2010s, the London Borough of Barnet Council, run by a Right-wing administration, felt it had come up with the logical answer: 'Not much'. Dubbed 'easyCouncil', its aim became to reduce itself to a handful of central staff, with almost every function outsourced: not just the services, but also the commissioning of those services. This reductionist approach proved deeply divisive and unpopular and led to leadership fall outs. The model was based on a view that the council had no role to play other than purchasing essential services: the council did not see itself as having any role to play as place shaper, leader or community builder.)

Regardless of the age or condition group of the person in question, success in health, care and a range of other public services looks something like the individual living both as independently and as socially as possible, with any health conditions or other risk factors well-managed by the individual and their family, with the support of experts where it is absolutely necessary. The purchaser/provider split, operating within a system with no mechanism for financially incentivising success of that kind, can result in both kinds of organisation feeling powerless and beholden to the other, and neither able to focus on what the people they exist to serve really want. Community-based providers are pressurised to offer the lowest unit cost support activities, regardless of long-term benefit. Hospitals operate within the nationally set NHS price-setting ('tariff') system, but this again pays for activities. Their economics require them to remain full and turning over patients rapidly above all else: empty beds are a financial problem. So is being too efficient:

the payment-for-rate-of-activity tariff system would mean that if, for instance, a hospital found a way of providing twice as many operations of a certain kind, their local commissioners, who have a limited amount of money to spend on those operations, could not allow them to do so. From the commissioners' point of view, there is no real 'market' of these large providers: the public service system they manage would collapse if their big providers went bust. A market in which organisations cannot go bust is not a real market. Commissioners also have no spare cash to fund innovation or the 'double running' costs of trying new things and there may be no real saving from local people becoming healthier (let alone happier), because all their providers have waiting lists of people waiting to fill vacant beds should more become free.

Most managers of commissioning and providing organisations genuinely want to improve things, but often fall back on 'transformation programmes', 'innovation' and 'efficiencies' which all add up to the only thing they can afford to do: cut costs. Even that cost-cutting turns out to be illusory as smaller, more stressed teams make mistakes or are unable to reach people who then experience even more disastrous – and expensive – crises.

In the face of the failure of the 'market' to innovate out of these vicious circles, central government has introduced waves of legislation, regulation and performance measurement in attempts to increase choice and quality while controlling or lowering prices. The Care Act 2014 set out a visionary purpose for adult social care: to enable people to achieve and maintain wellbeing, defined holistically to include a wide range of physical, mental and social measures. Councils were given new duties to have preventative interventions in place, to build their local market of providers and to offer everyone individual control of their care. But the economics of care remained unchanged, so the gap between that vision and what social care achieves widened. Councils maintained their freedom to spend their devolved budgets while the centrally set part of those budgets continued to be cut by up to 50% in some areas. The new duties were hard to enforce and unpoliced.

Central government tends to want to have it both ways, pointing to devolved spending powers when challenged on cuts, but also highlighting occasional modest (and un-ringfenced) remedial cash injections (such as the 'Better Care Fund') as evidence that it is putting money into the system. I have witnessed successive new social care ministers, their briefs seen as both politically toxic and subservient to greater good of the NHS, finding out just how little power they have to change anything at local level. Their best chance of making a difference would be to persuade the Treasury to part with more money for their unloved sector, but this is the task they find hardest to achieve.

Central government under Blair (1997–2007) attempted to introduce a dizzying array of performance management systems and targets, alongside its continuation of 'free-market' reforms, arguably ending up with the worst of both worlds. Targets were pared back significantly by the coalition and Conservative governments from 2010 onwards, partly on ideological, small-state, grounds but also drawing on evidence that many targets could be gamed and created perverse incentives. But with the 'market' no more functional and unprecedented budget cuts, NHS and social care performance declined against the available performance and satisfaction targets while social care improved on some measures but the number of failing services continued to grow.

In the face not only of competing organisations within a public service sector but also sectors themselves focused only on their own pressures and resources, some regulations attempt to penalise one part of the system for not working with the other. For instance, councils (who commission social care) can be fined if a lack of their services keeps older people in hospital when they are 'medically fit for discharge'. These regulations sometimes increase the adversarial nature of these inter-system relationships and create no new resources.

There have been some attempts to change how the money is spent and on what. Chapter Five will discuss the partial success of Direct Payments, which give a significant group of adults and families the option to take control of money which would otherwise be spent on their behalf. They have created a new kind of social care, but their numbers are limited. While a few areas help Direct Payment holders to form new groups and enterprises (the 'microenterprise' model discussed in Chapter Five), most find themselves as customers with limited means and a limited choice of imperfect services, rather than taking on commissioning power.

There have been attempts to change home care for older people so that instead of looking after them, with the risk that their own skills deteriorate, the approach is one of 'reablement', in which targeted support helps an individual build their strength, mobility and confidence. This is now routinely offered to many older people who leave hospital for a short period, but beyond this most UK home care remains unchanged, procured on price alone.

The economics of our public services need to change radically if they are to pay for the results we want. Neither monolithic centrally controlled bureaucracies nor 'free' markets have shown any real sign of achieving this, or wanting to do so. The models which most closely align to what people want are those which can operate at a human scale. The people most likely to design them are front-line workers and the people with whom they work. They will need a shared set of goals and rules within which to work and to be able to access a shared set of measuring tools to demonstrate their comparative success. Any sensible notion of 'good' in health and social care will value the capacity, connectivity and resilience of individuals, families and communities as much as the capacity of support services. This would require and result in some very different relationships between people who provide and people who need support. To enable this 'culture' change, we would need to embark on a shift in the way money moves, which would also require the one kind of change you cannot find discussed in any mainstream policy document: a shift in power.

Measuring the wrong things

Public service regulation is often characterised as red tape: bureaucracy which is a necessary (or at least unavoidable) evil. Many approaches to regulation are indeed bureaucratic, focusing like much else in public services on process: what can be documented and the validity of that documentation. But while having the right policies and procedures in place and records of them being followed may reduce the likelihood of abuse and certain kinds of failure, it says nothing about the actual experience of using the service. In fact, filling in the requisite paper trails inevitably takes practitioners away from the people they are employed to be with. It can feel more important to have recorded a risk assessment than to have thought carefully about all the risks facing an individual living within such bureaucracy. As a man who now lives outside of institutional care says of his time living in a residential home, "I couldn't go out to a club without having to do a risk assessment and care plan." Any trip out "involved a lot of planning ... for example how many staff and clients were going."

Care and health services are inspected by CQC, the government regulator. Inspections are vital in identifying failing services; without them, some of the worst abuses would remain undetected. But this can be after the fact: it is hard to detect and prevent poor and unsafe practice before it has happened. As outlined later, CQC has powers that in practice it is hard for it to use, and a limited role to advise on improvements. They can do little about the dangers caused by budget cuts. In some cases, failing and dangerous services have received clean inspections, as is inevitable in an imperfect and tightly resourced system.

Even with unannounced inspections, schools, hospitals and care services have been able to create an artificial impression for the inspectors. This happens in all regulated sectors: "When Ofsted come calling, loads and loads of schools hoover up the naughtiest kids before inspections".[1] A man with a learning disability described to me how in his care home, "The staff are much nicer and they don't boss you around when the inspectors are there."

This difficulty in getting behind some services' ability to create a facade, can lead to inspectors having a role which can be derided as 'turning up to count the bodies': an expensive way of confirming, too late, that a service has already failed. The Francis Inquiry into deaths at Mid Staffordshire Hospital Trust criticised inspectors' failure to prevent deaths and supported a switch away from a more collaborative inspection regime based on routine visits, towards a less trusting one: unplanned visits, with more thorough inspections targeted on services with risk factors such as patterns of complaints from patients. Some hospital inspections can now involve dozens of inspection staff and hundreds of days of combined inspector and service workers' time: in other words, workers' time and energy taken away from the people they support to liaise with the inspectors and millions of pounds of public money spent at a time when one of the key risks to safety in the services being inspected is the lack of public money to pay for enough front-line staff.

Some have argued that the future of regulation will be entirely data based: rather than inspectors calling, public services will collect sufficient data about the outcomes they achieve for people and people's views on their experiences, to create a real-time, multifaceted picture of performance which can be published live. Service managers would be easily challenged when their services fall below average or acceptable standards and could learn from those services which are producing the best performances.

There are problems with a data-based system of regulation however. Data is always gameable: as soon as data is collected and either measured by government or published, managers start to focus on making the changes which most improve their ratings and an industry springs up around achieving the best (apparent) results. So schools are accused of focusing most on those pupils who are near the boundaries between grades, because a small improvement or drop in their attainment will make a tangible difference to the school's performance, at the expense of those who are struggling most or could be achieving highest. The media regularly reports the experience of hospital patients who find themselves unattended in a corridor because they have been moved from one part of the hospital to another to avoid a waiting times target being missed.

A complete picture of a service needs to be coloured in by people's experiences of it. At present, people using health and care services are asked questions about their experience, such as the NHS's universal friends and family question: 'would you recommend this service to your friends and family', and there is some use of Patient Recorded Outcome Measures (PROMs), but these measures are a small part of a service's rating and services are not set up to find, hear and act on individuals' and families' feedback in a systematic way.

In fact, many services actively reject criticism from service users and relatives, regarding them as 'troublemakers'. A Competition and Markets Authority (CMA) report noted the widespread absence of consumer rights for the 'customers' of care homes and 'termination clauses' that are invoked to evict residents who have made complaints (CMA, 2017). Southern Health NHS Trust learning disability service 'aggressive[ly]' (Hattenstone, 2016) kept Connor Sparrowhawk's mother from being involved in his care before their negligence killed him. During a later tribunal it became apparent that Connor's mother's blog, in which she voiced concerns about her son's care, was seen as a major concern by professionals, with some having 'an irrational fear' of it (Ryan, 2017).

CQC now employs 'experts by experience', who have substantial experience of using services, in their inspections. Like many of the most promising reforms, this remains relatively small scale. While inspectors are well-paid employees of CQC, 'experts by experience' are sourced via third-party contracts and one contractor, Remploy, decided to cut their pay by 50% to the living wage and use zero-hours contracts, resulting in mass resignations of the experts.

The relative value of different people's opinions, and the power of those people to effect change, remains embedded in the adversarial inspection system: ultimately it is inspectors who wield power, not people who use services. Contrast this picture, and the very variable results it produces, with the situation of disabled people and families who take responsibility for hiring and firing their own support staff via taking a Direct Payment. Neither these unqualified, untrained and ostensibly 'vulnerable' people nor those who support them are subject to regulation, inspection or data collection, but there is no evidence that they experience greater risks or unhappiness; most report being more satisfied and happier.

What can we learn from them? We need data collection and recourse to inspections, but how much responsibility would we be willing to take on ourselves, for creating and maintaining an up-to-date picture of public services at those times when we find ourselves using them regularly, if it kept us or our relatives safer and happier? Is it possible that a more collaborative approach to keeping services safe and challenging them when they go wrong would not only be more effective, but would also reduce unnecessary cost and wasted time?

How research sustains failure

I have argued that while public services talk about achieving changes in people's lives ('outcomes'), they fail to organise their economics or regulations around this goal. One obvious way in which a public service can be focused more on outcomes, is to conduct research into the service and reshape it around 'what works'. A good example of a kind of support service that has moved from being haphazardly designed to being outcome-focused and evidenced, is the talking therapies which have become part of the Improving Access to Psychological Therapies (IAPT) programme, rolled out nationally as an evidence-based approach to providing easy-access support to the large section of the population which experiences low levels of depression, anxiety, OCD and other common psychological ailments. IAPT's expansion has been on the back of robust trials of the interventions it offers, such as cognitive behavioural therapy (CBT) (Hofmann et al, 2012) which has been demonstrated to be successful in relieving symptoms of mental distress after what can be a relatively brief intervention. It is undoubtedly positive that talking therapies are more widely available and that the ones which are offered have been researched and shown to be generally effective.

So the procurement of IAPT services usually has the common-sense goal to buy as many successful IAPT sessions for the least amount of money. An IAPT practitioner in an NHS service describes a packed work schedule with constant pressure from middle managers to move people through the service and close the case. The 'patient' fills in a feedback form after each session to track their mental health.

On the surface, this increases cost–effectiveness. But the evidence-based approach masks some problems. First, research shows that the quality of the relationship between therapist and client is crucial to the intervention's success from the client's perspective; a focus on client throughput can undermine that relationship.

The scales that patients are asked to use each time to score their mental state are well-researched but the IAPT practitioner says,

> People often tend to use the scales to say things are getting better because they are grateful and want to give you a good write up.

Furthermore, most mental ill-health symptoms can be linked to underlying issues: unprocessed psychological problems stemming from childhood, current relationship problems or stress and anxiety exacerbated by practical problems such as poverty and poor housing. A brief, highly prescribed intervention, cannot tackle underlying issues and without them being addressed, the individual might find symptoms repeatedly flaring up. Each time, they may be improved with a short course of sessions. This would look like success to the commissioners, despite being less cost-effective in the long-term than a more holistic approach, which would have to involve a range of different kinds of support and thus hard to manualise, research and measure.

So it is possible that positive results are being recorded for an intervention which may only play a small and tenuous part in someone's long-term wellbeing. If so, these records will in turn be used to strengthen the evidence base, giving commissioners more confidence in purchasing the service. A senior psychological therapist argues,

> The introduction [...] of the Improving Access to Psychological Therapies (IAPT) services has not brought the benefits it promised. Rather, it has imposed a limited model, with a limited choice of therapies, tight restrictions on the numbers of sessions and inflexible expectations of progress through treatment. (Boyles, 2017)

Whether CBT helps a lonely older person manage their depressive thoughts is measurable, but understanding how to tackle loneliness, how to help someone reconnect with old friends or make new ones, is complex and long term, which makes it hard to research. The interventions one would make into an individual's life to tackle the particular reasons for their isolation would need to be co-designed with the individual, rather than rigidly manualised. There are typically several different factors at play in success, it would be hard to pinpoint one cause for any good or bad effects and difficult or unethical to administer a 'placebo'.

There is research on those fields of practice which attempt to make less rigid, more personally tailored and more complex and long-term interventions into people's lives, such as the decades of research into what makes effective community development work. But those kinds of work take place more messily out in the community practised by charities more than by the state, and are rarely the subject of large robust trials.

So there is an inherently poor fit between 'rigorous' research and relational, holistic or complex interventions, and a commensurate good fit between research and short-term, medical interventions, which creates a self-reinforcing evidence and resource loop – a kind of academia/public service complex to misquote Eisenhower – which continually drives research resources, and then public service resources, towards medicalised interventions. Community interventions are caught in the opposing vicious circle of weak evidence leading to lower resources and vice-versa or they are obliged to adopt models such as IAPT designed by the statutory sector, 'abandoning the non-pathologising, accessible and flexible practices that meant their doors were open to the socially excluded' (Boyles, 2017). Given the diversity issues within academia, this is particularly so for research into BME-specific organisations, which tend to be smaller, locked in a loop of under-resourcing and exclusion from the groups which control resources. The National Institute for Health and Care Excellence (NICE), which decides which medicines the NHS buys and advises health and social care commissioners and providers on which kinds of support are well-evidenced, reifies these effects. Councils used to provide much more non-medical mental health support. Some of it, such as the day centre, was institutional (although often valued by some of the people using them), but there were also community-based support, outreach teams and funding for local charities and community groups which were often unique in being able to reach particular communities. Little was rigorously researched, but some was community work intended to address the underlying causes of people being disconnected in a way that the interventions currently being invested in do not attempt to do.

Just as the most powerful managers (that is, those with the biggest budgets and teams) are found in the largest, slowest to change services, so the most eminent researchers are those who win and direct large research projects into the status quo, not those who research small, innovative and disruptive services. I was once part of a panel sifting government research applications. The strongest applications on the scoring system were those which were most concerned with understanding current process and mapping existing services, because those research tasks are more easily undertaken and could generate quantitative data. The ones aiming to study more complex problems or emerging solutions were the most problematic to approve because any conclusions would be qualitative and open to challenge on cause and effect.

A typically 'evidence-based' approach to change involves small-scale 'pilot projects', which are evaluated over three years. The evaluation will usually find some evidence that the approach works for some people, but notes the small scale of the sample and calls for more research. The new approach may well appear to use public money more effectively (better outcomes or experiences for the same amount or less money) but it is very rarely possible for a small-scale initiative to demonstrate that there are any genuine savings to the taxpayer in a complex system of interrelated public services. Meanwhile, the special funding for the pilot has run out and there was no plan to transfer resources from mainstream services to the new initiative. The mainstream services continue to be regarded as non-ideal, with inspections and reports highlighting frequent failures, but they are where the resources are and they are a known quantity. So even though there is consensus that the hospital ward is not the ideal location for most healthcare, there is vastly more rigorous research into the factors that affect the quality of a ward than hard evidence to prove the kinds of community support that most reduce hospital admissions.

Rather than research driving radical change, research reluctantly follows innovation, with a lack of evidence routinely cited as the reason an innovation cannot be introduced. As the CEO of a large mental health charity, known for its innovative and effective, but patchily funded, community services said, "When it comes to evidence, we're ignored if we do and damned if we don't." The King's Fund (Gilburt, 2015) found that mental health service 'transformation programmes' were often simply the merger of previously specialist teams and increasing reliance on unqualified staff within medical settings and a range of 'community services,' which could refer to all kinds of support groups and activities with little discernible theory behind them, other than that they would be lower cost.

In recent years, a new breed of public services design agencies and 'labs' such as Nesta, have started to apply research thinking to designing new kinds of public service intervention. This has introduced deeper thinking about evidence, theories of change and cause and effect to innovations within public services, and has launched many new initiatives which can now demonstrate their cost-effectiveness and scalability, from Good Gym, which enables runners to (literally) run errands for isolated people, to Code Club, which has brought computer coding to pupils in 2,000 schools. However, even this more rigorous and better resourced approach has seen only a small number of innovations become embedded at scale within the health and care system, as those public services remain locked in to failure-sustaining economic models.

Why large services can fail but not fall

One of the fundamental tenets of any market, is that organisations which fail go bust and disappear. Your local hospital, however, will never go bust, no matter how badly it does. If you live in Mid Staffordshire, the Stafford Hospital, found to have killed perhaps hundreds of older people through poor care, is still your local hospital, just under the new name of the 'County Hospital', because the costs and consequences of letting it fall: of closing it and trying to start again, would be even more unthinkable than carelessly killing frail, older people.

Being 'too big to fail' can apply to the private sector as much as to the public sector. The Circle Hospital at Hinchingbrooke was an early and celebrated pioneer of attempts to introduce private healthcare providers. It was described as a staff-owned cooperative, although several years after it was founded, many staff at the hospital were not members of a cooperative in any legally recognisable form. The hospital had early successes in reducing its budget, followed by a well-publicised slide into financial difficulty, which resulted in Circle handing back its contract to the NHS with the hospital carrying a sizeable deficit. Like many hospitals and trusts before it, it was restructured and rebranded and business continued as usual.

In most markets, the failure and disappearance of unsuccessful organisations is a given. Entrepreneurs and their investors still carry on taking risks, because that is the only way to create the chance of success. In our public service systems, the impossibility of certain organisations being allowed to fail does not, as one might expect, create an environment in which it is easy to take risks, but instead, one in which it can be *impossible* to take risks. As budgets are ever more tightly squeezed, the largest, most expensive established services are prioritised for survival, leaving no resources which could be risked on even modest innovations.

A social care commissioner described to me one of the challenges he has in helping people to choose more effective and 'personalised' forms of care, such as Shared Lives, in place of traditional models of care, which generally take place in purpose-built buildings like care homes and hospitals. He recognises that people often live much better lives in Shared Lives and supported living and that Shared Lives in particular would cost him a lot less per person. This is partly because Shared Lives, described in Chapter Six, takes place in people's spare rooms rather than in a building which must be kept staffed and running to much the same standard whether it is full or half-empty. It would be better in the long term to empty the building and help people live in ordinary homes, but in the short term an empty bed would be a cost which he must carry. A gradual move towards a better alternative model would result in the current provision becoming gradually uneconomic. So zombie services remain hungry for the lives which feed their budget lines, long after they should have been buried.

In theory, one of the key roles of CQC is to close failing services. In reality, CQC has an extremely difficult decision to make when it encounters poor or even dangerous care. To shut a service down places additional pressure on the services that remain. Even a privately owned small care home may be home to 10 or 20 highly vulnerable older people, whose care is funded by the state. An inspector finding evidence of serious failings, such as verbal abuse of people with dementia, will be aware that for some frail older people, a move is as good as a death sentence. While CQC consistently finds that smaller care homes provide better care, it is these care homes that are closing most quickly during austerity. This is partly because, with no extra payments for successful care, their economics are harder to stack up, but perhaps also because, the larger the home, the more of a problem it would be for the local health economy and its commissioners if the home were to be closed.

Closure is not the only remedy open to CQC. Their inspections can, for instance, publicly label a service as requiring improvement or inadequate and for some kinds of service, it can enforce a 'special measures' regime of close supervision and enforced improvement. For a large NHS-run service this will be damaging to its reputation and staff morale, but it will also be accompanied by input from turn-around teams. For a privately owned care home, a rating of inadequate can in itself be tantamount to a closure notice, as both privately paying 'customers' and local council care buyers look for alternatives. The financial margins of running care homes are so tight that even a small loss of people needing support could bankrupt the owners.

CQC does use its powers despite their limitations. When it does so, it is vulnerable to lengthy and expensive challenges in the courts by providers trying to prove that its judgements were inaccurate. It cannot afford to run that risk too often. These factors help to entrench reliance on providers which no one believes offer the best possible care.

How could this be addressed? One way would be to abandon the idea of a market entirely and revert to entirely state-run care and health. To do so would be to forget that highly centralised public services tended to be highly impersonal and institutionalised; one reason why markets and choice were introduced in the first place.

Another would be to create a surplus of provision in the market, in order that there could be real choice and that poor services could fail with fewer deadly consequences for the people using them. It's hard to seeing this being politically and economically realistic. Instead, increasing scarcity is the prevailing trend.

As with the problems outlined earlier with public service economics and research, a third solution would be to change the location of power.

In both the private sector-dominated social care sector and the state-dominated healthcare sector, the people who use services, and their families, have the least power, while the bulk of the power is fought over by commissioners and providers in a dangerous game, like two children fighting over a bucket brim-full of scalding water.

Despite the introduction of individual budget control discussed in Chapter Five, most public services remain based on monopolies either buying care, providing it, or both. The same groups of people retain power no matter how badly local services fail. But what if the consequence of a care home or another kind of service failing was neither that a new team of outside 'experts' were brought in, nor that it disappeared, but that control over it was temporarily transferred to a trust run in the interests of people who lived in it, and with a board controlled by them, their families or chosen advocates. The management and staff team would find themselves, at least temporarily, answerable to people whose only interest was good, safe, effective care. This provision would have to be legislated for as a condition of entering the care market and the financial consequences would need to be undesirable, such as no profits removed from the organisation for the duration of its recovery.

Some 30,000 families collectively spent over £500 million a year on the huge Southern Cross care-home business which failed in 2011. Southern Cross axed 3,000 front-line support posts in the process of trying to stay afloat: as far as managers were concerned, the priority (and indeed their legally enforceable fiduciary duty) appeared to be salvaging the value of their shareholders' assets.

While the government and sector leaders debated how best to tackle the challenge of one of the largest care-home businesses collapsing, the voices of those 30,000 older people and their families were noticeably absent. No older person appears to have been made homeless as a result of the collapse, but many older people and families were distressed by the uncertainty. Presumably those 3,000 care staff had useful roles, so the impact of their dismissal will have been felt by those most in need of support. Certainly, the business's customers did not receive the best possible value for money for the £20,000 or so spent annually per person.

What else could such a large group have spent such a vast amount of money on, had even a small proportion of them been able to act as a group? Even a simple users' and families' group might have been able to influence government and the business owners in decisions which impacted on their care and security of tenure. But had some of those families been invited and supported to form a cooperative, they may have been able to wield their considerable collective buying power to very different ends.

Commentators on the sector predict more large care-business collapses and smaller businesses continue to go bust. What if we saw those collapses as opportunities for citizen-takeover of those businesses? Government loans could be used to purchase those businesses where enough residents, families and staff wanted to take them over. The property portfolio and the commitment of staff and families to using and improving the service would offset the risks of those loans. Offering groups of families first refusal on the purchase of the care businesses with which they had a long-term relationship could be legislated for, in much the same way that the *Localism Act 2011* enshrines communities' 'right to challenge' to take over struggling public services.

This approach of enforcing a temporary or permanent powershift where there was failure, would clearly discourage some kinds of organisation, particularly profit-motivated organisations, from entering care markets. This would be offset (assuming offsetting it was seen as desirable) only if, conversely, the financial consequences of really effective care which led to people regaining independence or experiencing fewer crises, were commensurately positive. In other words, a system of payments and interventions which rewarded success and punished failure, with 'success' and 'failure' seen as describing the achievement and maintenance of health and wellbeing by individual human beings.

The suggestions in this chapter will seem unthinkably radical or hopelessly naive to some. But without changes of this kind, we will continue to wish naively for more human-sized services which are more 'preventative', 'person centred' and 'community based', while continuing to resource those services that currently represent the biggest budgets, and which, while some achieve near-miracles when it comes to rescuing us from crises and medical emergencies, consistently fail to help us achieve resilient wellbeing and self-reliance.

A short guide to blaming other people

One of the most insidious ways in which institutions maintain their power to continue to fail is through their tendency to blame individuals for institutional failings. This is woven into public service language. For instance, 'bed blockers' are people who fail to be discharged from hospital quickly, but despite the term, this is hardly their fault. It happens when community services are not available or when hospitals and other services fail to work together well. Sometimes it is the individual or their family who are reluctant to allow their relative to leave the (perceived) safety of the hospital for home or a care home, and some staff report that a factor in this decision can be the fact that the hospital is always free under the NHS, while means-tested social care can be a large expense borne by the family. Mostly, though, the individual labelled as a bed blocker is keen to go home and their family are keen that this happens also, but they are victims of the stubborn lack of coordination and integration between social care and the NHS. 'Bed prisoners' would be a more apt term.

Another common term within medical care is the 'non-compliant' patient, who does not take the medication, or otherwise comply with their doctors' instructions. This reflects the parent/child nature of the doctor/patient relationship. I know that when I'm a patient, this can be attractive: I just want the experts to fix me and let me go. I am less keen to discuss any changes I need to make to live healthily in future. But this relationship does not work, particularly for people with long-term support needs who need to take medication, or adhere to certain diets or lifestyle changes for many years if they are to live well. If we design systems without talking to the people they are intended to support, we probably should not be surprised when those people are unwilling to fit themselves into those systems.

Sometimes, those systems are designed in such a way as to refuse entry to the people who need them most. But these people are not described as being failed, but as being 'inappropriate referrals'. A man with a mental health and substance misuse problem explained 'dual diagnosis' to a colleague: "Sometimes I'm drunk and mad, but at other times I'm mad and drunk." We have designed many of our interventions around a particular label, and built all of the structures of training courses, qualifications, clinical roles, funding streams and service specifications around those specialisms. We have done so knowing that many people with mental health problems self-medicate with substances, and that substance misuse problems can contribute to mental ill health. We have created few parenting support networks and resources which are accessible to parents with learning disabilities, but we are quick to decide that such parents will never be 'good enough'. We create children's and adults' services that cannot work together to help someone plan for adulthood, so that an individual's 18th birthday apparently comes as a complete surprise.

We cannot create specialist services for every possible combination of conditions, but we can recognise that whether people have one, two or more long-term conditions, they will generally have the same easily understood goals: to live well in a place of their choice, with people they love and something to do. If all services revolve around those universal goals, they can draw in the relevant expertise about particular needs or conditions as and when they are needed. This is only feasible if we were to share the responsibility for designing services that offer people the kinds of support, information, training and backup they need when they need it, and which allows people and families in turn to take back responsibility for their own lives.

This victim-blaming is not intentional: one of the mysteries of institutions and bureaucracies is that systems set up by caring, clever people, to help other people, often act in ways that have the opposite outcome to the outcome that everyone involved intends to have. There is lots of research into why people do not comply with medication or treatment regimes, but less into why systems don't comply with the intentions of the people working within them.

Much like a dystopian sci-fi film in which robots created to serve humankind develop their own ends and take power over their former masters, our public service bureaucracies can override the compassionate, humanising instincts of people who set out in careers to help others, and instead find themselves serving and ground down by 'the system'. They see that system as harmful, but feel completely powerless to change it. Feeling subject to something they do not see themselves as part of, they can only try to evade it, subvert it, or bend its rules.

It has been when they have let down people in their care that some organisations have been least able to accept responsibility, as illustrated by Southern Health NHS Trust's attacks on and attempts to 'manage' Connor Sparrowhawk's grieving mother in the immediate aftermath of his death (Ryan, 2014). At a time when humility and empathy were most called for, organisations have behaved in ways that make it hard to believe they are just large groups of (mainly deeply caring) humans. They have treated bereaved and angry families as communications risks to be managed.

Even in less tragic circumstances, you can see how organisations treat people who have good reason to complain without the respect and understanding that would be appropriate to any normal conversation between humans, while being quick to point out that the increasingly angry and frustrated individual is behaving 'inappropriately'. In another context, we expect people with learning disabilities to encounter the limitations of their support services without becoming 'challenging'.

What is 'appropriate' behaviour when we have been let down, had our dignity ignored, or even been bereaved? While all organisations must keep their teams safe and no one should go to work and face abuse, wise organisations recognise that, when it comes to these most personal and human situations of grief and anger, a group of 'professionals' acting within a bureaucracy may not be best placed to judge.

The ability and capacity to accept responsibility for services' failings, and a system which allows for humility, learning and apology, without those human instincts being routinely trumped by financial liability concerns or a scapegoating mentality, would be a key hallmark of a public service system that could move away from the demand for miracles and the pervading fear of failure, towards the expectation of qualified, 'good enough' success.

Escaping the invisible asylum: actions

1. New ideas of value
We need to ditch the idea that the value of our public services resides in buildings, kit, drugs or budgets. The value of a public service resides in the people who use and provide the service, the relationships between them and the health and wellbeing they create together.

2. No more 'pilots'
'Pilots' of new initiatives have failure designed into them: they ensure that we never have robust enough evidence to decommission large services in favour of small initiatives. Public money should only be invested with a plan for the gradual scaling up of what appears to work and the commensurate reduction in existing models which expensively achieve less.

3. Relocate power
The changes we most need to see are typically described as 'cultural'. In reality, they are changes in economics, regulation and knowledge. And behind all of those changes lies a change in who has the power within

our public services. While all front-line workers and people who use public services are excluded from sharing power and resources, people from minority groups and communities experience a further layer of exclusion.

FOUR

Risk aversion and risk indifference

Heavy Load was a punk band with five disabled and non-disabled members. As the film about the band showed (Rothwell, 2008) punks with learning disabilities may not even be able to live how and where they want, let alone throw TVs out of hotel-room windows. In one scene, one of the men is comprehensively overruled in his desire to move to a city where he hopes to live a slightly more rock and roll lifestyle, but where the professionals who have the final say on his decisions feel he may be unsupported or isolated. From the band and its punk ethos was born a charity called Stay Up Late, dedicated to helping people with learning disabilities 'fight for your right to party'. You may from time to time see an adult with a learning disability at a festival or a night out, but this will rarely be past about 7.30 pm. This isn't because they have to get to bed early, it is because support service shifts generally change over in the evening. The support worker has to get back in time for 'handover' to the night shift, so the person they support has to go home long before most nights out have even got going. Late nights out at rowdy venues serving alcohol can also be seen as risky, although the person being supported might be more concerned with the risk of missing out on fun and friends. Stay Up Late's neat solution to this is Gig Buddies, a scheme in which disabled and non-disabled people are matched around shared taste in music and go to gigs together. It is not a service: it is people coming together over a shared taste in music. While many support services have strap lines involving words like 'quality' and 'independence', Stay Up Late's motto is the best company motto ever: 'Keep It Punk'.

Earlier, I suggested that one of the signs that you are living in an invisible asylum is that you are in a place of 'safety', as defined by others who have a professional (but not necessarily personal) responsibility for keeping you 'safe'. The availability of support of this kind is a good thing: a society that lacks a 'safety net' will be one in which the times in our lives when we enjoy full autonomy are shadowed by the fear of certain kinds of illness, or simply of growing old (when one in three people born today will develop dementia (Lewis, 2015)). But it is important to recognise that support of this kind is never unproblematically benign. It is support which at times keeps people safe from death, but at other times keeps people 'safe' from life.

Societies repress marginalised groups by defining the risks they wish to take as transgressive, irrational or sick. A danger to themselves or others. Totalitarian regimes often hold their subjects in a stifling parental embrace. There may be a certain safety in this 'security'; a predictability which, for instance, some people living in former Soviet bloc countries reported missing when those authoritarian governments collapsed and left them subject to new economic forces and less predictable forms of power.

When your decision-making skills are deemed to be impaired by a condition such as dementia, autism or mental ill health, a complex legal framework kicks in which is intended to preserve your autonomy as far as possible, while also preventing you from taking decisions you are deemed incapable of understanding. This deprivation of full liberty from people who have committed no crime is a necessary evil that prevents, for instance, someone with bipolar disorder attempting to fly off a tall building. Few people with that illness, when well, would prefer to be given the freedom to make such a choice. Nevertheless, losing the freedom to take risks always entails losing one's full citizenship.

The *Mental Capacity Act 2005* and its accompanying regulations apply, for instance, when someone with dementia wishes to leave their care home but is not able to find their way about or to cross roads safely and so would be very likely to come to harm if allowed to do so. Rules cannot identify every set of circumstances in which someone lacks capacity to make a decision so broad concepts apply, such as working on a decision-by-decision basis (someone lacks capacity for a specific decision, they do not lack capacity in general) – starting with the assumption that an individual has, not lacks, capacity – and acting in a person's 'best interests'. There is always a degree of judgement and subjectivity.

Many professionals are very skilled and conscientious in supporting informed choice-making and risk-taking. But even the most skilled professionals have a finite amount of time and so necessarily base their decisions on a partial and subjective understanding of the individual and their wishes. This means that the extent to which people with cognitive impairments can exercise their citizenship depends not only on laws and regulations, but also on the resourcing of care and health services. A poorly trained or supervised worker, or one trying to cope with an unmanageable case load, will not be able to put the requisite time and energy into getting to know the individual and their circumstances well enough to make a good enough decision.

The actual degree of risk of an activity (even a mundane activity like visiting the shops) can depend heavily on the availability of support staff, so for some people the degree to which they can be full citizens depends also on a staffing rota, the adequacy of which can be traced back to a council procurement process and decisions taken about budgets by people who will never have direct contact with the people whose independence hinges on those decisions.

The Court of Protection in 2017 heard a case (Carson, 2017) in which, five years into their marriage, a couple were told by their local council that they must stop having sex, because the man, who had Down's Syndrome, had been deemed by a psychologist to lack mental capacity to consent. His wife would therefore have been committing a serious sexual offence had their marital relations continued. The remedy was sex education for the man, and the court case concerned a complaint that this education had not been provided for many months, during which the couple had moved into separate rooms in the man's parents' home where they lived and the woman 'significantly reduced any physical expressions of affection' to avoid 'lead[ing] him on'. Once 'educated', the man was then deemed to have the capacity for the couple to resume their sex life. Few other groups would have to fear a council or health official (not a court) criminalising their marriage. The judge felt the intrusion was 'lawful' and 'perhaps ... part of the inevitable price that must be paid to have a regime of effective safeguarding'; it was in his view the failure to resource the required remedy which inexcusably breached the couple's rights.

It would be interesting to know the rationale that led to a professional to decide that a married man was not able to consent to the 'committed monogamous and exclusive relationship' he had been in for five years with the support of his parents. Certainly, in many mental capacity cases, the attitude and creativity of professionals makes all the difference. Dementia Forward described their support for a keen runner, they nicknamed 'marathon man' who had lost contact with his running club as his dementia progressed at a relatively young age. His wife was having to hide the house keys and there was regular conflict as he wanted to go out running while she felt obliged to prevent him for his own safety. The charity found a volunteer who was also a runner and happy to go running with the man, which meant that the woman no longer had to restrict her husband's liberty to the same extent. Jill Quinn, Dementia Forward's director, told me:

> Marathon man didn't fit people's image of someone with dementia. His running friends probably either assumed he wouldn't be able to run any more, or weren't confident to offer their support. I used to use his story to recruit volunteers, but now my goal would be to support his running club to be inclusive.

While many large care businesses would be unlikely to have available staff with enough time, skills and motivation to understand the man's challenges from his perspective (I want to take part in my favourite hobby) rather than a service perspective (Mr X repeatedly tries to leave the house and becomes aggressive when staff intervene), this situation was resolvable because the people involved (the man's partner and a small local charity) were able to take a more personal and human perspective.

So risk-taking is an aspect of adult citizenship which can be eroded in later life by a combination of diminishing mental capacity, rigid application of rules and diminishing practical and social support to exercise what mental capacity we have. But risk-taking is also of course, a key aspect of growing into adulthood.

Growing into adulthood and independence inevitably involves some degree of conflict with our parents, whose ideas of what is practically or morally safe are informed by different times and experiences, and their own upbringing and temperament. Most families manage or at least recover from these conflicts, but they usually entail the kinds of behaviour (rows, raised voices, slammed doors) that exasperate parents but do not lead to consequences for teenagers and young adults which last much beyond being 'grounded' for a week or so.

Most of us do not really 'earn' our independence. We learn what our parents can teach us and from surviving the risks we take. Then we become independent, ready or not. Like many people, I look back on my early experiments with minor law-breaking, less minor drunkenness and poorly managed relationships with some shame and more wonder that I managed not to come to any real harm while I gradually became slightly less stupid. I hate thinking about my own children doing what I did, but I know that they will, and that if they don't make any mistakes, or take any risks, they will never truly grow up.

A young adult with a learning disability or another significant support need typically wants to take risks. They express anger in similarly 'inappropriate' ways to others. They learn life lessons, but may find those lessons harder to learn, including the lesson of how not to get caught. For many, a service or the state takes on a parental role at some point which can be when the young adult first leaves home to live in a service or supported tenancy.

This means that their progression to full adult citizenship is not a given. The more professionals, particularly medical professionals, are involved in their support, the more likely it is that risk-taking and conflict will be interpreted through the lens of pathologising psychological theories. The more concerns a service or professional has about an individual's ability to judge and take risks, the more their liberty is likely to be curtailed. For some young people with learning disabilities, this can in turn lead to greater frustration, more expressed anger and more verbally or even physically aggressive behaviour.

I have worked with young adults with learning disabilities who punch people when they are angry. It's not fun to be punched and as a professional at work you feel strongly (and correctly) that you shouldn't have to face fear or violence at work, no matter if that violence can be interpreted in the context of an individual's intellectual impairment. So support plans and risk assessments are drawn up. Medication is prescribed and even at times enforced. Progress is hoped for and small steps noted but, unlike most young adults, the young adult with a learning disability carries with them a detailed record of every 'incident' which is accessed by the ever-changing rota of staff who become intimately, but often briefly, involved with their lives.

Services run courses and support programmes to help people with learning disabilities to 'prepare' for independence or for entering or re-entering the community. To take such a course is as much about postponing independence as about bringing it forward. Young disabled people are already just as much a part of their community as anyone else; they should not need to pass an entrance exam.

In extreme cases, accounts of risky behaviour, whether real or perceived, can lead to lifelong restrictions for an individual. For instance, a young man who set fire to an object, later found to be associated with the abuse he was suffering, was still in secure accommodation years after any criminal sanction would have ended. Professionals reviewing his file and assessing whether he could 'safely' return to the community struggled to get past the word 'arson'.

The myth of risk aversion

It is commonplace to hear people in the long-term support business, when talking about how difficult it is to let people make the choices they might like to make, describe the organisations they work for as 'risk averse'. Large organisations being risk averse is another of the unavoidable, fact-of-life drawbacks of our current care and health system, but, although averseness to some very common risks associated with ordinary life is built in to the fabric of our current system, a closer look reveals that organisations labelled 'risk averse' are always, in fact, stunningly complacent to certain kinds of risk. So, like the other problems I have outlined in this book, dysfunctional attitudes to risk are not universal and inevitable: they are the results of choices.

If you look at the risks assessed and recorded by an organisation that supports disabled or older people, you will find that, while they are presented as risks for the person, they could equally be seen as risks for the organisation. In fact, the only risk assessment records you will find will be those which concern risks which affect the organisation as well as the individual. So you will find no risk assessments of the risks which worry people most, like loneliness, or failing to find a partner, although these risks particularly affect people with long-term support needs and are often increased by the very act of providing long-term support; it is hard to make and maintain social connections if you live in a care home, spend your days in a day centre, or must organise your life around support visits and hospital appointments. Service buildings are often closed to the outside community or physically distant from it and in some parents and relatives are kept at arm's length and consigned to visiting hours. This separation between service and the rest of the community is not only isolating; it increases the vulnerability of people who rely entirely on a staff team member being willing to 'break ranks' and whistle-blow, if something goes wrong.

A participant at a social care conference in 2014 described how her organisation had explored supporting its service users, who have learning disabilities, to date. They found a dating agency, Stars in the Sky, which specialises in working exclusively with people with learning disabilities and has many more safety features than a typical agency. The decision the organisation made, however, was that this posed too great a safeguarding risk. The worker was clearly experienced, compassionate and well-motivated; she described the decision and the 'risk averse' nature of the organisation she worked for with regret: one woman she supported had said that her main life goal was to find a boyfriend.

The risk was described as a safeguarding risk to the individual, but safeguarding is not typically a risk that we put first when attempting to pursue love or a sex life. The really unacceptable risks were the financial and reputational risks to the organisation, should the woman experience harm. Even with all the support and advice available to her and the use of a specialist dating service, the young woman could not be viewed as being able to take any responsibility for pursuing a sexual relationship, so the organisation supporting her felt obliged to take all the responsibility themselves. She may be more likely to suffer serious harm getting the bus to college or crossing a busy road, but an accident on the roads would not attract the attention of something going wrong following use of a dating site, perhaps because many people remain uncomfortable with the idea of an adult with a learning disability wanting a sexual relationship in the first place.

We have some sense of how many older people living in care homes suffer from poor care, or abuse, but not of how many are lonely, although a large international study concluded that lacking social connections is a comparable risk factor for early death as smoking 15 cigarettes a day, and is worse for us than well-known risk factors such as obesity and physical inactivity (Holt-Lunstad et al, 2010). This is a particular risk for older people. The CentreForum's 2014 report *Ageing Alone* (Kempton and Tomlin, 2014) shows that nearly half of over-85s admit to experiencing loneliness some or most of the time and highlights research showing that one in ten people visit their GP because they are lonely. However, few services would recognise those risks and almost none know how to respond to them.

So organisations are not risk averse, but risk-selective: highly averse to some risks but breathtakingly complacent about others, including, shockingly, the risks they themselves cause. Attempts to eliminate the perceived risks create new ones: the widespread insistence of support services on police-checking everyone with any contact with a disabled person creates the risk of friendlessness.

It is legitimate to consider the risks affecting an organisation you work for or manage, but we also have a duty to consider the risks we create and if we are given an individual's money, or public money spent on their behalf, shouldn't we think of them all first from the point of view of the individual?

Do no harm (unless you measure it)

Ignoring risks that the service itself causes or exacerbates is an example of how, where public services measure 'outcomes' at all, they only see one kind of outcome: positive ones. Most professionals will recognise that it is also possible for a service to have a negative outcome, but there are no tools in widespread use in any service sector that are designed to measure such a thing. In fact, the whole concept of negative outcomes of good services is almost entirely missing from policy thinking, practice guidance, commissioning plans, care and support plans, research and evaluation. Negative outcomes are only recognised or highlighted where a service or professional is seen to be failing in some way, and then the harm is uncovered during an inspection or emergency review of some kind. For instance, an inspection may uncover concerns, or a manager recognise that an 'unboundaried' worker has 'fostered dependence' in their 'client', through making the mistake of being seen to offer friendship, or even love, when it is their proper role to maintain professional distance and neutrality.[1]

And yet, almost every service intervention can have negative outcomes as well as positive outcomes. When it comes to medicines, we are used to this idea and the risk of side effects. Being fully informed of the side effects is a crucial part of weighing up whether to take the medicine and doctors see it as a basic good practice to discuss them with their patients. This kind of discussion never occurs when someone is offered a long-term support service. In fact, most practitioners would be nonplussed were the individual to whom they were offering support to ask, 'What are the side effects? What are the risks of this intervention?'

Partly this reflects the lack of real theory or evidence sitting behind the manuals, policies and procedures of most support interventions. It is assumed that support interventions do good, but practitioners and managers would for the most part have to think hard in order to articulate the cause and effect chain between their interventions and the good which is hoped for, and would draw a complete blank if asked for the evidence of that theory of change. In this evidence and theory vacuum, discussions about services become hopelessly polarised and ideological: services are 'outdated' or 'modernised'; people are either 'attacking' or 'defending' them.

This is not to argue that no long-term support services 'work'. A home-care service that results in an otherwise immobile older person getting up, dressed and fed every morning has a self-evidently positive impact. But if that older person, until recently, got themselves up, dressed and fed, it is possible for some that they might do so again with the right – probably complex – combination of support, motivation and challenge. And few home-care services are constructed around carefully thought-through or evidenced approaches to slowing deterioration in independence or rebuilding independent living skills. Support to maintain or restart life as a social citizen is usually completely absent. A care home where there is support and physical safety may be a more beneficial place to be than at home with periods of no support, but those benefits are not weighed against the inevitable harm done when one is taken from one's own familiar surroundings, relieved of all responsibility and separated from social and family contacts. The care homes which have a clear aim to maintain skills and social relationships are few.

Research can tell us something about the kinds of support approaches which often work for particular groups of people (for instance, older people recovering from stroke as opposed to older people with dementia), or in response to different support needs or situations (for instance, older people on their own, as opposed to older people living with a partner), but traditional research is unlikely to offer a full answer to the question of what the overall balance of benefits and disbenefits is of a particular service, or how to maximise the positive balance. The 'correct' (or more realistically, good enough) answer to that question must also be informed by the individual's own views and that of their family, because each situation is unique to the individual's state of mind, attitude, fears and beliefs, and is constantly changing. This complex view of what would be the best support is hopelessly out of kilter with many long-term support services that are delivered by unqualified workers paid little more than minimum wage. But the costs of getting the intervention even slightly wrong are huge, not only to services but much more importantly to the individual, as both become locked into a pattern of ever greater intervention and ever greater presenting need.

Too much support can prevent a physically impaired individual from building or rebuilding their physical strength or dexterity, or their confidence and mental aptitude, to take charge of everyday tasks, resulting in a support need that will occur several times daily for the rest of their lives. These real costs and opportunity costs[2] are that much greater if the individual relies exclusively on such services for their wellbeing.

While there is evidence on the physical impact of receiving support on frail older people, there is little research into negative side effects that support services can have on a person's relationships, including their relationships with family carers or other 'informal' sources of support, despite this being a key part of nearly every individual's ability to live well independently. Some of the ways this happens should be visible: building-based services physically remove people from family and community relationships (sometimes replacing them with new sets of relationships formed within that building, but which, again, are often not thought about and valued, as can be seen when day centres close and people are not supported to continue to socialise with the friends they made there). Some of the ways this happens are invisible: being labelled with certain conditions or support needs is stigmatising and encourages people to avoid the person labelled as being mentally unwell, for instance. Many services operate inflexible schedules or have fixed opening times and some require extensive travel to reach. Even home-based services purchased with personal budgets may be inflexible, as reports into home care for older people have highlighted, requiring individuals to rise, eat or go to bed at antisocial times, as noted earlier in the book. Services do not offer to adjust their schedules to fit around an individual's social activities or family routines, thus making them harder to maintain.

Community care law was set up to recognise people as individuals only, not as part of family units. Assessments and care plans were produced on an individual basis, regardless of the interdependence of one family member's routines, support needs, goals and wellbeing on their partner, child or relatives. This has been particularly felt in the inability of social care support for adults to support those adults in any parenting role they may have[3] (Wates, 2002), resulting in parents being seen as incapable (when with the right support they were entirely able to parent) and children being forced into inappropriate caring roles (Aldridge et al, 1998; Aldridge and Becker, 2003). The *Care Act 2014* attempts to address this, through mandating and encouraging the option of whole-family assessments and plans, if people want them, and the promotion of the recognition and support of family carers and young carers, but support services that are able to respond in this whole-family way have been slow to develop, and parenting support services slow to become accessible to disabled people and other parents who have their own health or support needs.

It is not just the complexity of measuring the positive and negative whole-person or whole-family impacts that stops it happening. Our unconscious belief system, in which professionals have responsibilities and agency, while 'patients', 'clients' and 'customers' have 'presenting needs' to be met, is incompatible with seeing individuals as people who have pasts, relationships, the desire to be responsible citizens and long-term futures and goals. With this world view, relationships and families are complications that get in the way of the high-pressure, poorly resourced work of large support services. In hospitals, day centres and care homes, outsiders can seem to the staff team like disruptions to their work to be minimised and managed. A visitor can be a huge boost to the wellbeing of someone confined to a hospital bed and families (particularly families of people with dementia or other conditions that result in someone becoming distressed in a place they don't recognise) often describe providing hands-on support to their relative in lieu of hard-pressed ward staff. But many hospitals operate visiting hours and control visiting from the perspective of the risks posed by people accessing wards unchallenged, rather than balancing that with the need to enable access for family carers where that is needed.

If measuring long-term support services' side effects became the norm, the relative success of different models of care, and the relative success of 'formal' and 'informal' care, would have to be reassessed. Some would fear that highlighting the potential harm done by services, particularly by those not already well thought of, would just add to the current wave of attacks on the efficacy of public services, which have coincided with a political drive to reduce the size of the state through spending cuts and privatisation. That risk is undeniable but, conversely, it is only through a more careful description of the benefits and limitations of public service support that public services can be properly valued and investment in them justified.

Redefining responsibility and how to share it

If we are to end the pervasive culture of selective risk aversion that pervades our public services, we will need to take a very different – much fuller – view of risk. We cannot change our view of risk without first changing our view of responsibility.

Having responsibility – being held responsible by others for what we do (and fail to do) – is the defining characteristic of being an adult and a citizen. Becoming an adult feels at the time like it is a fight for rights and freedoms, but – surprise! – it turns out to be a battle which we have won when we find we have responsibilities. A place of our own becomes a rent agreement or a mortgage; the freedom to spend money as we wish becomes the responsibility to earn it and pay bills; the freedom to have sexual relationships becomes the responsibilities of homemaking and, for many, child-rearing. As we age, particularly in Western countries, we gradually divest ourselves of these responsibilities: children grow up and leave home (eventually), mortgages are paid off (we hope) and we retire from our jobs (perhaps). If we develop support needs, we give up our remaining responsibilities.[4]

JRF research over five years consistently found that even older people with high support needs valued being able to keep friends, make new ones and remain active citizens. Being able to contribute, as well as receive care, was important to wellbeing, but to professionals older people with high support needs 'are still largely perceived as people "in need of support" who need to be "taken care of" – rather than as citizens with rights, responsibilities and contributions to make' (Bowers et al, 2011: 5; see also Bowers, 2009; Bowers et al, 2013; Blood, 2013).

One of the least-heard pleas of older people with high support needs is, 'I feel useless'. Moving to a model that JRF describes as being based more on reciprocity and mutuality, could, therefore, have significant positive impacts on health and wellbeing, perhaps extending healthy lifespan and reducing or delaying the need for more intensive support. Replacing traditional home care, which simply maintains an older person by doing for them those basic self-care tasks which they cannot do themselves, with a 'reablement' home-care approach, as described earlier, goes some way towards this goal, through encouraging self-care, but stops short of recognising the health-giving potential of enabling older people to socialise and help others.

The process of unlearning single-direction support (and the commensurate dependence) can be uncomfortable for both worker and the person they support, even if the end results are positive. Even the switch from task-oriented home care to independence-focused reablement can result in older people report feeling less well cared for, as they find doing tasks that were previously done for them initially tiring and stressful. For some, simply regaining the physical ability to get up, get dressed and prepare food, and perhaps the mobility to use buses or taxis, may be enough to become a part of their community again. For others, the barriers are much more deeply rooted: lost confidence, lost relationships (due to distance or death), lost roles and a lack of accessible community activities and roles. So, it would be a much more ambitious shift to adopt the goal of older people regaining or building a social life, being and feeling 'useful'. A handful of initiatives have shown that this is possible, however, often through taking an intergenerational approach, such as the Homeshare approach discussed in Chapter Eight, in which an older person with a spare room offers accommodation and in some cases, mentoring, to a younger person, who helps out with physical household tasks, or the Dutch and now UK examples of co-locating nurseries within older people's care homes or day centres, to the obvious benefit of both age groups.

While older people may lose some or all of their responsibilities towards the end of life, for many people with significant long-term physical impairments, learning disabilities or mental health problems, responsibility may be rarely or never experienced, despite the desirability of social relationships and employment, volunteering or other meaningful activity being accepted as a key part of wellbeing and enshrined in legislation and accepted within all the relevant strategies. Numerous large-scale studies have shown that friendships, employment and other forms of responsibility are correlated with increased physical and mental health (Waddell and Burton, 2006; Holt-Lunstad et al, 2010). But rates of employment for disabled people and people with mental ill health remain low and achieving them is low down services' priorities and often regarded as 'too difficult'.

A key reason for this is that we conceive 'responsibility' in narrow terms; largely, monetary terms: is our balance sheet of money we contribute to the state through taxes, and money we gain from the state through service costs and welfare benefits, in the red or the black? Politically, this is a highly toxic issue. The Right tends to combine a distaste for anyone requiring significant state support, a lack of empathy with those who cannot avoid doing so and a lack of trust in the ability of the state or its services to do anything other than foster dependence. The Left tends to see any discussion of responsibilities as code for cuts and combines this with an unquestioning belief in the benevolence of well-funded state interventions. So in slightly different ways, both Left and Right see responsibility in financial terms and neither have confidence in the capabilities and potential of people who need support.

Direct Payments (discussed in the next chapter) involve an individual with a support need being given the money instead of the service for which that money would previously have paid. The individual or their nominated family member (theoretically) has greater rights to choose the nature of their support and (certainly) more responsibility for managing it. For some critics, particularly on the Left, this would or has led to more self-interest, undermining, rather than increasing, people's sense of responsibility to each other, although there is little evidence to support this and to the contrary, many small groups of people who use services and of family carers have used their new access to resources and the confidence they have gained from controlling resources to collectivise in ways that have had a profoundly positive effect on state services. This can be seen particularly in the rise of hundreds of user-led organisations that provide support to disabled people to live independently, scores of self-advocacy organisations that enable people with learning disabilities to have their voices heard and hundreds of tiny social enterprises started by small groups of people who use support, and their families.

So there is evidence that people will, when they can see how to, take more responsibility for their own care and also in some cases, form lasting relationships and alliances. These initiatives happen on a small scale, with the result that they have been easily dismissed as insignificant, or resisted as a messy 'fracturing' of previously stable, large services. But it is only on a small and personal scale that people with support needs are able genuinely to begin to take on and exercise personal responsibility. In recent years, even small groups have access to the mass communication technologies that give them the opportunity to form alliances between themselves. This makes possible individuals and small groups starting to coordinate their campaigning, decision making and resource managing power on a much larger scale, built from the ground up, rather than designed centrally, which would always mitigate the extent to which any responsibility sharing is genuine and taken on willingly and on people's own terms.

Escaping the invisible asylum: actions

1. Seek out and take the right risks

When a public service or one of its workers manages or avoids a risk they perceive in someone's life, too often they ignore a whole series of risks inherent in their intervention. There is risk inherent in every human interaction. Risk is as necessary as oxygen. Organisations that are 'risk averse' are in fact blasé about the risks – loneliness, dependence, lack of freedom – that matter most to people: it is only the risks that matter most to the organisation to which they are averse. If you are not helping people to understand and take risks, you are preventing them from living.

2. Measure your harm

Even great services create harm; they will become better for seeing and measuring this harm. Organisations need an approach to things going wrong which is agreed in advance between service, staff, individuals and families, and which includes a frank discussion of what risks the individual wants to take, the support they need to do so, and how responsibility will be shared on the occasions when things go wrong.

FIVE

The humanisation experiment

My only friends in life are my paid carers.
(Carter, 2016)

England's adult social care system has seen one of the most concerted and long-standing attempts at radical reform of a national public service in the Western world. Called 'personalisation', a term that never gained widespread understanding, it could be described as the attempt to 'humanise' the long-term support of disabled adults and to a lesser extent, older people.

Social care, which revolves around ongoing personal care and practical support for adults who either live in their own homes, or who live in service buildings such as care homes, is perhaps the least well understood public service. Most UK citizens, if they have any concept of it, believe, wrongly that it is part of the freely available NHS, and are stunned to find (usually at a point of family crisis as an elderly relative develops ongoing support needs, perhaps following a fall, stroke or dementia diagnosis), that their life savings and inheritance might be needed to fund care which in too many cases is both expensive and very basic. While most UK voters are deeply suspicious of any privately run provision in the NHS, they have not noticed that most adult social care has been privatised over many years, nor that this was followed by an even more radical set of reforms, giving people, in theory, complete control over the money spent supporting them. The thinking behind these reforms is now quietly being introduced for up to 100,000 NHS patients and is even being explored in sectors like criminal justice with little history of valuing its key ideas of choice, control and community living.

So, this humanisation experiment is worth understanding. It also shares many of the aims of the new health and care model that I will set out in the second half of this book. And it was a partially successful experiment, demonstrating both what is possible and what, so far, was not.

Putting people first

A key goal for social care in the 1990s was to close the hundreds of large, long-stay institutions for disabled adults and people with mental health problems, which were widely recognised as failing to offer people the opportunity of pursuing ordinary life goals, as well as having been exposed as harbouring high levels of abuse and poor practice by the Griffiths Reports from 1988 into the 1990s. For decades, parents were encouraged to give up their children to state care which was for many a system of 'warehousing' individuals considered less than human, with little or no potential and few rights. Many staff tried their best to be humane, but nevertheless abuse and misery were rife. Meanwhile the social model of disability argued from as early as the 1960s that what 'disables' people is not primarily a physical or intellectual impairment, but society, through its physical inaccessibility to people with mobility problems, its negative attitudes and prejudices, and communities' tendency to exclude (Oliver et al, 1983).

In the 1990s Person Centred Care focused on developing an individual picture of a person, particularly with a focus on their support needs, and developing an individually tailored care plan. Large numbers of people moved out of large institutions and into much smaller care homes, often based in ordinary family-sized houses. While some of the worst excesses of institutionalisation were eradicated, there was no strong evidence that people were consistently achieving the goals in their person-centred plans. Resources were still being allocated to individuals by professionals in processes that excluded individuals and their families and that were based on the costs of a narrow range of professionally controlled interventions.

Like Person Centred Care, Self-Directed Support was developed in the UK by In Control and other organisations, drawing on the US and Canadian work of John O'Brien, Connie Lyle O'Brien, Beth Mount and others (O'Brien, 1989; O'Brien and O'Brien, 1988; Mount, 1992). It was the idea that individuals and their natural support networks were best placed to be the experts in their own lives and support needs, had more potential to think creatively and take positive risks than professionals, and needed to be the key decision-makers about their own support and lives if they were to become and be seen as full citizens. These developments were primarily driven by activists who were working-age disabled adults and the families of people with learning disabilities. The new approaches in theory applied to the care of older people, but in reality were seldom adopted by older people's support systems; a gap in ambition which persists today.

Direct Payments – the right to take and control the cash equivalent of a social care service offered to you – were enshrined in UK law in 1996. Their roots were in US-inspired disability activism including Project 1981, the 'escape committee' of five disabled residents of a residential care home who in 1979 set themselves the goal of moving into ordinary homes. One of them, John Evans, achieved that move with council funding, for the first time (Brindle, 2008).

With a Direct Payment, someone who previously had to accept the support offered to them by their council, however poorly it fitted with their lives and aspirations, could now demand the money instead, and in many cases start to hire and fire their own support staff, resulting, for some, in a level of control and independence unheard of previously. However, take-up remained very low as local councils declined to promote them widely and many disabled people and families were daunted by the challenge of becoming legally responsible for employing their own support teams.

The broader concept of the personal budget was intended to make personal control over state budgets more widely accessible. People who have been assessed (or in some cases, have self-assessed) as eligible for a service are told how much money is available to fund their service and are given the option of taking control of that money, either through taking a cash Direct Payment as before, or through asking their council or another organisation to spend the money for them on their agreed support goals. From 2010, family carers and other 'Suitable Persons' could take on the legal responsibilities of managing and spending a Direct Payment on behalf of an individual who lacks capacity to do so.

Personal budgets were adopted as a fundamental delivery method for social care in 2007, when a 'concordat', *Putting People First* (HM Government, 2007) set out four radical changes, which drew on the broader concept of 'personalisation' developed by Charlie Leadbeater (Leadbeater, 2004):

- Individuals having choice and control over their services through personal budgets.
- Widely available low-level support to help people avoid a debilitating crisis.
- Universal access to the information needed to make new choices and plan.
- Work to building more inclusive and supportive communities ('social capital' or 'community capacity').

It was these four linked but very diverse changes that became known as 'personalisation': an attempt not just to change how services were organised or paid for, but also to change how a much wider group of people interacted and thought about services (so that fewer would need formal services at all) and even to change the nature of communities when it came to their interaction with their disabled and older citizens.

In the subsequent years, progress was most in evidence for only the first of these four changes. Many councils have reported for some time that they offer every adult they support a personal budget. Although in some areas this simply meant a letter asking people if they were happy with the service they were receiving or wanted to change it, around 130,000 people have (harder to fake) cash Direct Payments (NHS Digital, 2016) and have used this new power to create a new workforce of directly employed Personal Assistants (PAs) which make up nearly a quarter of the 1.6 million strong social care workforce (Skills for Care, 2012) The outcomes and wellbeing of Direct Payment holders are, on average, significantly better than for other groups (Hatton and

Waters, 2014), with some disabled people able to become fully active citizens for the first time. Hiring and firing their own staff, rather than accepting a succession of strangers assigned to them by a large agency, has transformed people's lives, enabling them to pursue work, a social life and family relationships. The jobs created are often also more rewarding than the rushed and pared-down roles within many care agencies. As one wheelchair user and now professional disability consultant put it recently, "My PAs stay for years, because we form a bond and they enjoy the role. It's give and take on both sides."

There is also likely to be a significant gain to the overall public purse when people who might previously have relied on state benefits and services for every area of their life, are now able to organise their own care, to pursue a more active and included lifestyle and in some cases to gain employment. As one individual put it to me, "Employing a PA doesn't just mean I can get better support, it gave me the confidence to start my own business and I take more part in my family and my community."

In theory, personal budgets can be spent on anything that meets the needs identified in an individual's care plan. While adults with physical impairments are most likely to spend their personal budget on a PA, adults with learning disabilities or mental health problems and older adults are more likely to buy another kind of support service, with significant percentages of all groups spending their budget on community or leisure services, and a small proportion buying equipment or mobility aids. People whose main issue is isolation (perhaps as a contributing factor to a serious mental health problem, or as a consequence of struggling to make friends due to a learning disability) have spent their budgets on season tickets to football clubs and contributing to the petrol costs of a fellow fan who can help them attend. Others have pursued their dreams of training for a particular career or have started new community groups with their peers.

Despite these successes for self-directed support, the wider idea of personalisation has remained deeply contested, with critics arguing that it is a form of privatisation that undermines the idea of collective responsibility and the welfare state, or a way to disguise budget cuts (Needham and Glasby, 2014). The evidence base for its impact relies heavily on surveys and has been criticised for its gaps and weakness (Burkett et al, 2016). Many people working in social care struggle to describe it beyond the idea of personal budgets. Before outlining a new model of health and care support, it is worth considering what personalisation achieved, what it couldn't change, and why it remains so controversial.

First, it is important to note that, in contrast with some in both the Conservative and New Labour governments who presided over the changes, the people who introduced individual choice and control did not believe in a simple free-market view of public services, in which giving individual service 'consumers' choice would drive innovation, competition and better value for money. That could feasibly work where people need to buy health-related kit (there is a healthy market in spectacles for instance, which benefits both those spending their own money and people who receive NHS funding), but buying long-term support and the relationships inherent in that support is very different. Alongside more individual choice and control, the other three changes in *Putting People First* were regarded as equally important to ensuring that not only would services change, but also people's lives and communities. Those three changes were still little in evidence by 2014, when the new *Care Act* enshrined personal budgets in law and attempted to address the unfinished business of prevention, information provision and building communities.

One reason the impact of personalisation remains contested is simply that it did not happen, at least not evenly, for all groups. While a quarter of social service users have a Direct Payment, most councils are reducing their spending on prevention and non-critical services, have far from universal information offers, and remain unable or unwilling to take on the role of community builder. This was true before the 2008 global crash but during the ensuing austerity, in which some councils have seen their government funding halved, the disparity between deteriorating local spending and the national vision for personalised social care and healthcare is almost Orwellian: cuts to services are routinely dressed up in the language of empowerment and independent living. Building-based services such as day centres are incompatible with most people's ideas of personally tailored community living, but when those services are closed with little idea of what will replace them, following 'consultations' which are clearly a foregone conclusion, the rhetoric of independence, empowerment and community rings hollow and mutual mistrust grows between people who use services and people who provide them.

Even the offer of individual choice and control is much less in evidence than the legal rights to it would suggest. The offer of personal budgets and Direct Payments makes sense only if people who need support are trusted to take better decisions than professionals, but social care remains guarded by the 'gatekeepers' of scarce resources who require people to undergo needs assessments, eligibility tests and means tests which can be summarised as requiring individuals to prove they are sufficiently in crisis, sick or disabled and poor, before they can engage with planning processes intended to promote independence and creativity (Fox et al, 2013).

Extreme austerity is exacerbating a paradox at the heart of the personal budget concept, which starts with giving people an estimated 'upfront allocation' of money, so that they can make realistic plans. The chicken-and-egg challenge in this is that, to plan your care, you need to know at least roughly how much money you are planning with, but this amount is largely determined by how much your care will cost, which depends on how to choose to spend it. This has always meant that many areas work on the assumption that people with personal budgets will want to spend them on traditional care models or PAs, and estimate their allocation based on the hourly rates of that limited range of models, thus starting the planning process with a lack of creativity. 'Resource Allocation Systems', designed to generate this estimated allocation to aid planning, morphed into ever more bureaucratic systems used to constrain budgets, with their algorithmically generated figures treated as the final budget allocation rather than the helpful estimates they were supposed to be. Now, during austerity, the amounts people are allocated are reducing rapidly, with the consequent decrease in affordable choices and increase in the need to battle against the system, rather than plan collaboratively.

Direct Payments and personal budgets were a deliberate disruption to a public service system which was reluctant to let people take control over their lives. They are a transfer of power, in its monetary form. But disrupting the status quo is not easy, particularly when you are marginalised and may have difficulty communicating or leaving the house unaided. Bureaucracies are in fact designed to remain stable, consistent and predictable, which means that they inevitably resist disruption.

So while the majority of social care users report slowly increasing choice and control, in 2011, 26% of disabled people reported that they did not 'frequently' have choice and control in their lives, a slight increase on 2008 (Department for Work and Pensions, 2013). The BBC *Panorama* exposé of abuse of people with learning disabilities at the Winterbourne View Assessment and Treatment Centre in 2011 brought to light the existence of more than 3,000 people with learning disabilities who were living, in some cases for many years, in hospital-style and institutional facilities, more than half of which failed the subsequent programme of inspections (CQC, 2012) and little evidence of progress towards independence. Many were excluded entirely from self-directed support by virtue of being in the medical rather than social care system. It took a high-profile government-backed change programme longer than six years to achieve even a modest reduction in the use of this broken medical model.

Some groups have historically made less use of personal budgets. Only 29% of eligible people with mental health problems have taken up a personal budget, compared to 83% of people with learning disabilities. People from minority communities have lower uptake of personal budgets (and in mental health are over-represented as recipients of more coercive forms of treatment), which is in keeping with a broader pattern of health access inequalities (Moriarty, 2014).

Personal-budget uptake for older people, people with physical impairments and family carers all stand at 64% (NHS Digital, 2014). Some have concluded that choice and control over care are therefore not important or attractive to older people: what older people want is someone to organise efficiently good-quality care packages, not the stress of choosing between numerous providers during a crisis.

It could equally be observed that choice is not an end goal for any group; it is only positive in as much as it is a means to achieving a better or more personally tailored service. So while some working-age disabled adults who have stable entitlements to significant resources have been able to exercise choice and control to design and control their own care via PAs, older people typically have small or non-existent allocations of state funding, with fewer able to afford a team of PAs (only a quarter use their personal budget in this way (Burkett et al, 2016)). Their needs may be as much social as practical and there has been little development of affordable, tailored new care services designed to help them stay active, social and connected. Instead, a personal budget for an older person and their family might simply mean choosing from a list of care providers all offering an increasingly pared-down version of the traditional home-care service model that would previously have been purchased by the council. This group is much more likely than working-age adults to use a personal budget on a traditional care and support service and less likely to access a community or leisure service (Burkett et al, 2016).

The service offers designed for disabled adults have been designed in the context of a significant shift in attitudes: disabled children are more likely to be educated in mainstream education, people with learning disabilities who would have lived in institutions are living in their own flats and even getting married, disabled people and their families have formed vocal movements that have seen their rights enshrined in law; more recently Paralympic sport and various TV programmes have challenged attitudes. Meanwhile attitudes to very elderly people have not obviously changed; as dementia has become more common, the perception of older people as incapable has perhaps hardened. This perhaps helps to explain the lack of imagination in older people's services: large 'care homes', some of them with corridors of box-like bedrooms with no resemblance to 'home', are still seen as acceptable and even economically inevitable for the last years of our lives, while the regulator has refused permission to build care homes for younger disabled adults with more than six or ten bedrooms, because they would be too institutional (Turner, 2017). While families of disabled adults have usually had years to adjust to their roles as negotiators and advocates, and there is an advocacy sector (albeit an underfunded one) dedicated to helping them make good choices, older people and their families tend to have thought little about social care before making a 'stress purchase' of care in the aftermath of a crisis such as a fall or diagnosis and are poorly placed to shop around, let alone redesign a service.

If 'choice and control' really means less of the same, with added responsibility for managing money and contracts, it is unsurprising that older people have remained unconvinced. In contrast to the mainly state-funded support for working-age disabled adults, a great deal of older people's support is paid for by the older people themselves; they already in effect have personal budgets and the freedom to spend them how they wish. But beyond the development of hotel-style care homes at the 'luxury' end of the market, this purchasing power has not led to improved services or radically changed models. What power there is remains with the providers, while individuals can spend £20,000 plus a year on a small bedroom in an institution staffed by minimum-wage staff rotas.

Contrasting the experiences of Direct Payment holders, who have created and control a new model of care, with those of older people, who spend large amounts of their own money on often disappointing care, illustrates that the changes envisioned as 'personalisation' cannot be reduced to mechanistic changes in the movement of money. For personal control over budgets to have an impact, it is necessary either that individuals can design a whole new kind of service themselves (as Direct Payment holders have done in inventing the PA), or that the state or another body develops new kinds of provider from which people can choose. Even then, if the route to getting a personal budget remains one that is difficult and demeaning, with an inadequate or unstable care budget as the goal, people again lack the power to create real change. A number of different kinds of change must happen at once, which makes this kind of whole-system change rare and the impact of its individual parts difficult to evaluate.[1]

The patchy way in which reforms have been realised means that even within low-uptake groups there are nevertheless pockets of humanised approaches. For instance, hundreds of older people with dementia access family-based Shared Lives day support and short breaks in place of day centres and respite in care homes. Dementia Adventure is a social enterprise offering older people and their partners or families supported outdoor activities with an emphasis on fun rather than care. Even within the most 'traditional' sectors, there are examples of radically humanised thinking. Some care homes for older people are building links with their local community through, for instance, inviting community members to use gardens previously given over to lawn as allotments, while others invite residents to take on roles such as meeting and greeting visitors, in response to residents saying they wanted to contribute, despite their high support needs or low mobility.

The elusive 'community'

People with mental health problems are another group that has been slower to use Direct Payments, despite being among those who stand to benefit most from such approaches (Forder et al, 2012; Bennett, 2014; TLAP et al, 2014). For this group, barriers to change have included the traditionally medicalised culture of mental health services that have been slow to buy into the idea of patients, rather than clinicians, as experts and tends to focus on the real and perceived risks associated with diagnoses. Mental illness is a condition that both grows and feeds off isolation and part of its remedy so often lies in other people.

The Centre for Social Justice, in a 2011 report on mental health (Callan, 2011), argues that the move from institutionally based mental-health support to 'care in the community' has failed in many respects, because there was no commensurate focus on the community development work needed to ensure that 'the community' was welcoming and supportive for people with mental health problems and other support needs. There has been a tendency to regard community as a location, rather than recognising that it is a set of relationships. Many of the prevailing assumptions behind professionally led support have remained unchanged even while that support has been moved from large purpose-built buildings to smaller buildings, including ordinary houses.

On the 12th November 2015 the BBC's *Today* programme reported the upsetting and at times surreal story of a man in his 60s undergoing an acute mental health crisis in which he started to self-harm and become suicidal. His family were left to cope as best they could until they felt their only option was acute care. They had to call an ambulance, but instead of taking their relative to hospital, the ambulance crew had been instructed to take him to a 'mental health café' which could offer a cup of tea and a chat. As the man's daughter pointed out, they had tea and chats at home: they were looking for emergency care. However, this care had become more tightly rationed (cut) and instead the local NHS Trust was trying to rely more on 'community' solutions. The man and ambulance crew sat outside the café, which he was too ill to go into, for two hours, before the crew decided to ignore their instructions and take him to the Emergency Department. Eventually a bed was found and he spent several months intensively supervised in hospital.

The CQC's 2016 report on crisis care found that only 14% of people who experienced a crisis felt that the care they received provided the right response and helped to resolve their crisis (CQC, 2016). Meanwhile, more people are being 'sectioned', with a quarter of junior staff in one survey saying they were told it was the only way now to get access to hospital. Where they fail to do this, overstretched community teams are asked to visit people who need round-the-clock support, which may be leading to higher suicide rates.

Leading health researchers The King's Fund argued that, 'Despite the lack of guidance and evidence, most trusts have embarked on transformation programmes at scale and pace with little or no dedicated funding for the process. Arguably this has resulted in trusts taking a leap in the dark.'[2] We should, though, be cautious about concluding that moving mental health services from hospital to community is always an error and that a hospital ward is the only or best place for people to recover their mental health. The detail of the King's Fund report (Gilburt, 2015) paints a picture, not of acute services being closed and the money reinvested in 'the community', but of resources available to both hospitals and the family or community being cut, with no attempt to maximise the value of either, much less to coordinate them. The language of 'transformation' and 'community' care was being appropriated to a traditional cuts and mergers programme. There was no investment of training, support and emergency backup for the family carers who make up many unwell individuals' immediate communities. The family in the BBC report were providing round-the-clock emergency care to a very ill relative, but their only access to backup was to call the emergency services.

The BBC report is a nice illustration of the choice we are often presented with: keep all the money wrapped up in hospitals, or see them cut and an ambulance may arrive to take you for a spot of basket weaving when you are in the middle of a full-blown psychotic breakdown. There are small-scale examples of successful, humanised approaches to supporting people's mental health, such as 'men's shed' projects in which older men at risk of isolation social while using and sharing skills such as woodworking. Some medically based mental health services are supporting patients to become their staff's trainers.[3] Social prescribing allows GPs to 'prescribe' access to community or leisure activities to isolated or lonely people.

But 30 years after the advent of community care, it is time our public services invested seriously in finding and building community. This quest does not start at the national level: society may be 'big',[4] but community is small and personal. The internet age has seen breakneck pace development in how we connect with each other (and become isolated from each other), but while social media companies invest billions in virtual communities, we are yet to see any significant investment from government in our communities: how we find them, build them and rebuild them.

The power of small groups

While much of the thinking around personalisation focused on helping people to be seen and to act as individuals (rather than part of a homogenous group), a little noticed but potentially transformative movement made possible by that individualised approach has involved people choosing not to interact with their services as isolated consumers, but to form small groups of like-minded people.

Pulp Friction looks nothing like a public service. It was inspired by an experience Jessie Carter and her mum Jill had in 2008 when they saw a smoothie bar at a local festival in which static bikes powered the smoothie blenders. Jessie, aged 16 at the time, had wanted a part-time job in a restaurant or café like others her age, but she was finding that goal hard to achieve. Jill had the idea for the community interest company (CIC: a type of not-for-profit enterprise) of which Jessie is now a director. Pulp Friction enables young adults with learning disabilities to run their bikes at different community events around the country. The young people develop social and work-readiness skills. It has a small paid team that includes people with a learning disability as well as a team of disabled and non-disabled volunteers. Jill says, "Every time people buy a smoothie from us they are interacting with someone with learning difficulties, and that is really what Pulp Friction is all about – people-connecting." From this quirky beginning, the CIC is now running the canteen at Nottinghamshire Fire and Rescue Services HQ and a museum, and has been approached to do the same thing for two other agencies.

Co-founder and director of DanceSyndrome, Jen Blackwell, always had a passion for dance, but as someone with Down's Syndrome found it hard to find suitable training and performance opportunities. With support from her family, she formed her own company in 2009. Disabled and non-disabled people work and dance alongside each other in workshops and performances. Jen won the Enterprise Vision Inspirational Woman of the Year Award for the North West. Jen's Mum, Sue says,

> It's difficult to get across the enormity of Jen's journey with DanceSyndrome. After ten years of fruitless searching for training for Jen to become a dance leader, we realised we would have to create what we needed. As the enterprise grew, it would have been easy to hand over the reins, but the leadership has to remain with the dancers with learning disabilities.

There are now hundreds of enterprises like – that is, completely unlike – these two. Community Catalysts is a community support organisation that has a network of over 600 enterprises.[5] When it starts working in an area, Community Catalysts will find up to 80 small enterprises that are contributing to care and health in the area but which are completely unknown to the state or even the voluntary sector.

It is easy to regard them as most 'serious' policy makers have done: lovely, but tiny and unreplicable, and therefore to be talked of wistfully, but of no real consequence in the big picture of public service funding crises and reform programmes.

This is a mistake. Microenterprises demonstrate what is possible when people bring their own resources – time, favours from family, friends and neighbours, links to local businesses and in many cases their own money – together with state resources, usually in the form of Direct Payments. The results can be put in terms that public services can understand (people living more independently, moving towards or into employment, volunteering, being part of communities) but often can't deliver. The most common argument against giving control of resources to people and families is that they will act selfishly. They will maximise their own support, be profligate or simply incompetent. In fact, instances of fraud and waste remain rare, but the creativity and solidarity of small groups of people can achieve far better value for money than traditional care businesses.

One of the positive changes during the personalisation era is the rise of user-led organisations (often called self-advocacy organisations where the members have learning disabilities), in which people using services (and/or their families) have varying degrees of control, such as forming a majority on the board of trustees or directors. Many ULOs are used by councils and health trusts as part of their consultation processes and they enable the voices of people who use services to be heard by those who control them. The rapid growth of ULOs is a tangible demonstration of powershifting since the advent of personalisation. It is also an illustration of the limits of that power shift so far: most ULOs are haphazardly funded through the intervention of locally powerful people and that funding can end when that person moves on to another post. Almost none are a core part of the delivery of hands-on care, which would attract large and stable shares of health and care budgets. Their numbers are tumbling during austerity.

Rights without responsibilities?

ULOs and self-advocacy organisations are an example of people organising together to take the rights to which they should be entitled. They have now hit a glass ceiling, not just because current power structures are reluctant to offer them further rights, but also, more insidiously, because people currently in positions of power find it hard to see how they could share their responsibilities with such groups.

I was a guest at a meeting of Partners in Policymaking, a grass-roots network of people using services (family carers and their allies), whose members discussed the impact of cuts, as felt in the changed behaviour of care managers who were reducing vital support packages. This was a group of parents who had everything to lose and fear, but rather than being dominated by anger, the group quickly recognised that the people making decisions which they felt were having a profound effect on their lives, were, nevertheless, human. There was a discussion about what led to well-motivated people who had chosen caring professions to act in ways which didn't reflect their innate values. Two mothers argued that rather than anger, compassion and empathy towards those professionals was perhaps more powerful. This was not a case of 'letting them off the hook' for 'just following orders', but recognition that the people they were in conflict with felt as trapped by the lack of resources and the systems within which they worked as they did. One mother felt that she had a *responsibility* to be empathetic. Insisting on empathy as the most important value in service relationships felt like a subtle but powerful challenge to the prevailing culture of hard-nosed accountancy at the top, passed down through bullying into cuts at the front line, met with angry – but ultimately ineffectual – protest by families. The mother was not, I think, giving up her right to be angry and to demand change, but powerfully assuming a share of the responsibility to care for the people who collectively lacked the power to care for her and her child.

The relatively weak (for most) forces of individual resource control rain harmlessly on the walls of service structures, which are rotting in the way a concrete tower block rots: quickly uninhabitable but still standing in disrepair decades later. Deep changes to the beliefs and ethos of services are often described as 'culture changes'. But when leaders talk of wanting a culture change, they are generally describing changes which they don't feel are entirely their responsibility to make, and which they believe are unlikely to happen. In fact, most changes described as 'cultural' are, if they were to happen, changes not in culture but in power. Personalisation was an attempt to shift power by creating new rights to control money. However, genuine power changes are not simply changes in people's rights: rights are always an illusion if they don't entail a commensurate transfer in responsibilities. The promise of rights, without recognition of how responsibilities were and could be shared differently, was a limitation in the transformative ambition and impact of personalisation.

Tiny on a massive scale?

Research (Hall et al, 2014; Needham and Carr, 2015) into the impact of their size on the ability of services to tailor themselves to individuals tentatively suggested that very small enterprises may have greater potential to align themselves with people's lives and to form close relationships with communities. (These are benefits which the charity sector as a whole claims as its unique selling point, but which large national charities may in fact struggle to achieve if they become unmoored from the communities they are intended to represent.)

Not all micro-scale agencies are quite so uncategorisable as Pulp Friction and DanceSyndrome. Many are simply very small-scale versions of familiar services, which point to the possibility of redefining public service sectors that we know are dying. A single Community Catalyst in Somerset supported 170 micro-scale home-care enterprises, in which 180 mainly self-employed individuals offer paid home-care support to 600 older people in their village or area. Rather than rushing from visit to visit for an agency which extracts a significant chunk of the money older people pay, these people market themselves directly through parish magazines, libraries or word of mouth. They get paid more per hour than agency workers, while offering older people more time and a more personal and flexible service. This has dramatically increased the home care available to families in a rural area which large agencies can find uneconomic. Replicated nationally, this modest initiative would support almost 100,000 older people: collectively much larger than the largest home-care business.

Other initiatives have seen people develop small-scale day activities to replace large day centres and food businesses in which neighbours replace impersonal tinfoil-tray meals-on-wheels franchises, including one council initiative in which older people were offered a personal meals budget and a broker who helped them source the meals of their choice from local food businesses, who welcomed the older person to their premises when they could make it, and delivered when they could not. Either way, those café or curry house proprietors also became part of the older person's social network and early warning systems if the older person was not seen. Some of these enterprises, founded by people from BME communities, have tailored their approach to food, activities or support to a particular group or community in ways which larger agencies have not.

Each of these kinds of initiative has several things in common: they start with people's assets such as their creativity or ability to cook; they build local marketplaces rather than rely on a notional free market; they broker personal relationships but have some backup in place if things go wrong; they keep local money local, rather than it drain out of the area towards shareholders. Through enabling people to contribute more and to share responsibility, they also increase people's status and open a path towards achieving rights that traditional support cannot unlock. The people involved are closer to becoming commissioners, who design services, than many who use their personal budgets in more recognised ways.

The scale of these microenterprise approaches is currently very modest, but it has been achieved within a system which is designed for large organisations. Sometimes this results in rules which are diametrically opposed to the success of innovators and start-ups, such as the area that requires all its home-care providers to have in place electronic swipe-card systems: pointless and prohibitively expensive to providers which send the same person from their tiny team every day. Other areas undermine their promotion of Direct Payments and personal budgets by insisting that any provider on which state money is spent has several years of council contracting under its belt, effectively banning innovators and start-ups. A few web-based start-ups have attempted, so far with limited results, to use technology to enable self-employed people to offer their support and to match them with people who need support. While large numbers of us feel confident in our own ability to choose a minicab or overnight accommodation through an app such as Uber or Airbnb, we are understandably more cautious about choosing an intimate care worker for an older relative in this way and government agencies are yet to explore if it is possible to develop social care recruitment, assessment, care-planning and regulation to enable this to be done with confidence.

So it remains easy to conflate the necessarily micro-scale of the individual enterprises with the currently small scale of the sector as a whole. Growth so far has been in an unhelpful climate where neither local nor national government have demonstrated any real ambition for scale. Like many of the most promising public service initiatives, they remain the preserve of entrepreneurs and mavericks, who will always, through sheer determination, chisel a space for themselves in the most unforgiving environments.

The problem of scale is the conundrum at the heart of reforming long-term support services. We want human interactions, which can only take place at the scale of family and community. But we need this to happen affordably for millions of people and with enough consistency to ensure that gains for some are not matched by abuse and neglect for others. Little is yet known of the economics, risks and potential of humanised public services if we made them the core of our long-term support approaches. This would be as profound a change for public services as the move from institutions to community care.

It would be analogous to the communications shift from print and broadcast media to social media.

Imagine we need to design the way that humans get their hair cut. There are millions of non-bald people. Between them, UK people grow 150,000 metres of hair a year, weighing 12,000 tonnes (I am making these statistics up). There are hundreds of different hairstyles. Hair cutting involves using sharp and sometimes very hot implements, millimetres from people's heads and eyes. Apply a traditional public service design ethos to tackling this hair tsunami: the only way to balance practicality, safety and affordability would be to offer a series of large contracts for out-of-town hair cutting centres. To keep contracting costs low, these contracts would be large. Successful contractors would swallow up smaller ones. Some prime contractors might subcontract to smaller, specialist voluntary sector haircut providers. Minimum quality and safety standards would be maintained by government inspectors.

In reality of course, the hair cutting industry is dominated by tens of thousands tiny one-shop operations – microenterprises – that operate with little regulation. Most people can find a hair stylist whom they like and trust. Despite the warning from *Sweeney Todd*, barber industry scandals are few. Could the future of small, personal care and support be a range of tiny local organisations from which to choose, rather than being a customer of a large, distant, shareholder-focused business? Or to pick up on my earlier point, perhaps the organising principles we are looking for have something in common with the social media and sharing applications which most of us have allowed into the most intimate recesses of our social lives.

Despite the success which many people have made of unregulated Direct Payment-funded support, I am not arguing that we replace our highly organised public services with a free-for-all for all people. Many of us benefit from a structure or template in which people with health or support needs can interact with people with certain knowledge, skills and qualifications. We may need independent third parties to act as advisors, advocates and a recourse for complaints. But the examples given earlier show that people can meet safely and successfully within a much less rigid and oppressive framework than they do at present. We will never invent a risk-free system, but with different structures and relationships would things go more wrong more infrequently and more right, more frequently?

From this swirling and fractured history of personalisation, we can draw some clear conclusions. It *is* possible to humanise services, including the most medical and traditional. Given the resources, some people with long-term support needs (or their families) *can* create new models which fit better with their lives. But for some, control over money makes no difference, because the power differential between them and the services they need remains too great. While some of those who have created the most successful support arrangements are, unsurprisingly, educated, confident, articulate and middle-class, many others cannot translate their theoretical right to make choices into creativity or control, without the support of a specialist advocacy or brokerage organisation, which are scattered and often poorly funded.

Holding a personal budget in many cases has raised an individual's status from 'service user' to 'customer', but has not resulted in the status of 'manager' or 'commissioner', much less 'mentor' or 'leader'. As one parent who manages a personal budget on behalf of his son put it, 'This morning we had the review of the Personal Budget ... It was the usual stuff of extraordinary controlling behaviour and total lack of understanding of the life of the person receiving the budget or of the person they're expecting to manage the budget' (Neary, 2014). And even where someone has been able to choose (or even help design) a better support service, this doesn't always add up to a good life, which relies on things that money cannot buy, like friends, purpose and love.

Small numbers of individuals and front-line workers will always rebel against even the most oppressive and wrongheaded bureaucracies, but their actions will remain the exception rather than the rule for as long as the system and its power structures remain unbroken. So personalisation was and remains a fraught but necessary attempt to change the power dynamic between services that hold resources and people who need to use them.

Escaping the invisible asylum: actions

1. Scale down, scale out
Our public service system is full of large, inhuman services which need to scale down. Meanwhile, the successes of individuals who hold personal budgets and small, human-scale enterprises do not need scaling up to become the new problem, but 'scaling out' through creating the conditions in which many more people can make real choices and take their share of power, resources, knowledge and responsibility.

2. A good life is better than a good service
If you are using public services long term it can be hard to step back from the constant battle for support to ask:
• What would a good enough life look like for me and my household?
• What am I (are we) willing to do to get there?
• What do we need from services and others?
Enlist as many people who care about you as you can identify in asking and answering those questions. There are organisations which can help with this.

3. Connect
Building personal connections within our communities when we are well is like saving money for a rainy day: no one ever regrets it. And every council and NHS trust should have a long-term investment strategy for its communities (which will outlast even the most expensive buildings). While we believe the only resource available to a public service is money, our public services will remain bankrupt. We need to look for, value and ask to work with all the local charities, social enterprises and community groups that can reach local people, including those from communities routinely shut out of current discussions, who in turn can help to design and deliver better interventions and better places.

SIX

Shared Lives

Paul moved in with Shared Lives carer Sheila and her husband just before his fiftieth birthday. Sheila helped Paul to get a bus pass, to learn to use public transport and about road safety. Paul started to access dental services to address long-standing dental health issues, which has improved his overall health and bought his first bicycle, biking with Sheila and her husband to the countryside. He joined several clubs and got to know shopkeepers, library staff and even bus-drivers. Sheila encouraged everyone to 'look out for Paul' whenever he is out and about in the community on his own. Paul doesn't have a lot of speech, but when asked if he understands what 'independence' means, he smiles and says 'walk'.

(Story provided by Birmingham Shared Lives Scheme, 2015)

The first half of this book outlines why I believe that nearly every aspect of how we design, fund, deliver and monitor public services for adults who need long-term support is flawed, and how our public service culture remains steeped in the thinking that once built prison-like institutions. It chips away at compassion, which is the very reason good people decide to dedicate their working lives to helping others, and at the capacity and potential of the increasing number of families living with one or more long-term conditions. Meanwhile the media and half-informed politicians rant about failure from the sidelines, while big business licks its lips.

That critique is only of value if there is a realistic alternative. There is plenty of agreement about what must be done: we need to integrate services, innovate, focus on outcomes, share best practice, value the workforce and shift resources to prevention. All could be true, but all are exactly what public service managers have tried to do for decades without success.

It is also important to say that the immediate crisis in health, care and other services would be mitigated through committing a greater percentage of our GDP to them. Following the 2008 crash, two governments shrank the relative size of the state for long-term, ideological (as well as short-term, economic) reasons. An injection of public money would reduce the current crisis, but we have no reason to believe it would end it. The problems outlined in this book became entrenched during the boom years, when public spending was increasing as rapidly as it is decreasing now. In any case, that upward spending trajectory could never match the demographics-fuelled curve of public service cost. Something was always going to have to give. Specifically, it is in our long-term support services that the intractable problems of both cost and outcome lie, and it is on reform of these kinds of support service which the second half of this book will focus.

The dehumanising effect of long-term support services is talked and written about by disability rights activists, families and charities. Service 'reforms' are written about by think tanks, policy makers and economists. The subjects are treated as if unrelated. The purpose of this book is twofold: to make visible the root causes of failures in long-term support offered by public services, which are not those usually identified by commentators and politicians, and to set out a sustainable alternative.

What would an alternative long-term support system look like if it was humanised, but also operated at national scale, with workable systems and economics? It would have to feel entirely personal to people involved, while being applicable UK-wide, in small villages and huge, multicultural cities. It would have to be capable of supporting people with significant, complex and lifelong physical or mental health conditions safely and to do so at a significantly lower cost than current services. It would draw on unpaid family care, volunteering and the naturally occurring resources of communities, alongside the expertise, money, training, backup and infrastructure of services, with those different kinds of resources amplifying each other, not competing or clashing. Many of its services would occupy a strangely liminal space: formal but embedded within community. The support they offered would build people's confidence and capabilities, without abandoning them when they fall. This would be a more human system but also one which demanded more of us all. I think we are ready for it, because it already exists, in almost every area of the UK. It remains little known and underutilised, despite repeatedly demonstrating both affordability and staggering success in tackling exactly those human-shaped challenges which baffle and bankrupt our dehumanised services.

This book and the ideas of public service reform it outlines are drawn from my contact with the people involved in the Shared Lives and Homeshare sectors. Having started my career in the front line of traditional social care, my more recent years in these non-traditional sectors have given me a new lens through which to see institutional cultures previously invisible to me. The journey I have made under the influence of their shocking, entirely natural attitude to life and care is the journey I wanted this book to embody. I am not proposing that Shared Lives or any other approach is industrialised and imposed as the next great public service hope. There is no single model that everyone wants: real choices are essential. But Shared Lives could be offered to many thousands more people and even more importantly, its core approaches could be applied to every long-term support service.

Shared Lives is so humanised most people who notice it – and indeed some who live within a Shared Lives household – do not realise it is a service. Behind those ordinary-seeming households lies a largely unobtrusive infrastructure: the government's care regulators have constructed an inspection regime that avoids intruding in people's lives but does not sacrifice safety: CQC consistently says that Shared Lives is safer and performs better in its inspections than every other form of regulated care. This is not bought through spending more money: Shared Lives is significantly cheaper than traditional models. It has already achieved a national scale and rapid growth in social care for adults with learning disabilities, mental health problems, dementia and other conditions, and has now started to put down roots in health, criminal justice, family support and even domestic violence responses.

Its success suggests that other smaller initiatives, such as Homeshare and the community enterprises mentioned in Chapter Five, could scale from their current niches to become the core of a very different kind of public service system, with other, more traditional, services taking on some key aspects of their practices and ethos. We need to find an affordable way to humanise all of our long-term support services, without sacrificing the safety and consistency that we look for from them. The 'personalisation' reforms in the previous chapter showed us that partial reforms have patchy results. Shared Lives offers an ethos that could be universally applied.

Talk to one of the UK's 10,000-plus Shared Lives carers and they typically say that the person who lives with them or visits them regularly is 'just part of the family'. That individual is likely to be an adult with a learning disability but can also be someone with a significant, long-term mental health problem, or another support need such as dementia, frailty due to old age or a physical or sensory impairment. Shared Lives carer Jean says: "People say, 'You must be a saint', but I don't see it like that. It just comes naturally and I think I get as much out of it as she does. She's just one of the family." Rose says that Ben "brings life into my home as soon as he arrives. He always has a smile and is so easy-going and relaxed. We both love music and singing and we both love getting the most out of life. It's a pleasure."

Shared Lives takes the model of family care for disabled people and others with long-term support needs, which is provided by over 6 million Britons, and creates the conditions in which people choose to offer that level of support to someone from outside their family. This starts with a 'matching process', by which people who need support and approved Shared Lives carers are introduced to each other, gradually spending more time together before deciding on whether they are a good match. It should only be when both parties feel that there is a match that any long-term support arrangement is established.

Half of the 14,000 supported people live with their chosen Shared Lives carer as part of the family. Some of them do this for a short time during a crisis such as illness or hospital discharge or as a stepping stone to getting their own place, via which they can learn independent living skills and build the supportive relationships they will need to live well by themselves. A quarter of people use Shared Lives for short overnight breaks and another quarter for daytime support. For these people, the episodes of care may be shorter, but still regular and taking place long-term. Many Shared Lives arrangements and relationships are lifelong: I regularly meet people who have lived together for 30 or 40 years and intend to live together for ever, and people with learning disabilities who are now living with the grown-up son or daughter of their original Shared Lives carer, after than individual has retired from active caring.

Those long-term or lifelong arrangements draw not just on the caring skills of the trained and paid Shared Lives carer, but on countless hours of time spent with family and friends, who consider themselves to be neither working, nor volunteering, but spending time with someone they have grown to love. That longevity runs counter to public service culture. Most services are judged on throughput of 'cases', with little attempt to measure long-term outcomes. Shared Lives carers often have to argue against the assumption that the goal for every individual is to 'progress through the service' to 'greater independence'. That goal is right for some people, but Jean says of the person she supports, "She has lived in lots of services. She wants somewhere to settle." Several Shared Lives carers have told me that the person who lives with them gets anxious about visits from social workers because they fear being told they must leave.

There is much support and informal time which is unpaid within Shared Lives, but Shared Lives carers are not volunteers: they are paid. While there are many examples of 'gig-economy' care workers, who are tightly scheduled and controlled by managers, Shared Lives carers (when local organisations follow the national model) are genuinely self-employed: they work with the people they choose in their own homes and with a great deal of flexibility and autonomy. They are not paid by the hour and do not work shifts, although their payment should be commensurate to the level of support they are expected to provide and they should not be called on to provide 24/7 hands-on care. There is the risk of exploitation, but good local Shared Lives schemes recognise that the quality and longevity of the relationships within Shared Lives are the reason it works and is lower cost: twisting the model into a conventional 'service' quickly becomes a false economy.

By devolving more decision making to the household level, people are able to achieve unexpected things. When the organisation I work for surveyed our members about things people did for the first time in their lives through Shared Lives, they talked about people who had never previously looked anyone in the eye, or who had been entirely non-verbal, 'unfurling', 'blossoming' and 'finding a voice'. They talked about achievements which meant a great deal to them but which typical services either did not consider or considered too difficult or risky:

> One of our housemates has had his art etched on the glass walls of a newly renovated crypt at Rochester Cathedral – and he is soon to embark on his first solo exhibition ... aged 70! (Sarah, Shared Lives carer)

> P told us his lifelong dream was having a tattoo of Bruce Lee. He was always told he was not allowed because he has a learning disability. We had to do a capacity assessment, but P now has his tattoo and is walking on air and showing everyone proudly. He is 76 years old. (Shared Lives carer)

One young man with a learning disability passed his driving test. Others obtained their first job or joined a club not exclusively for disabled people for the first time. These achievements, which were out of reach to expensive services and highly trained professionals, were often achieved through support from people in Shared Lives households who have no qualifications, experience or professional status, but who see someone as part of the family: "[He has] learnt how to ride a bike for the first time ever. This was mainly through our children encouraging him."

Niamh, aged 12, described the people who visit her household for short breaks:

Even though Sam is blind he has got a great sense of hearing and never misses a trick! At first I thought me and Sam had nothing in common but I was wrong, he loves music and I love music. We have lots in common so when Sam comes to stay with us on a weekend, at night I go on YouTube on my laptop with him, he says which songs he wants to listen to and I find them for him which he then listens to on his headphones – this can go on for hours! My friends have become a big part of Shared Lives because whenever they come to my house in a morning to meet me for school and someone's been stopping the previous night, they always say 'hello' and 'how are you?' (Fox, 2015)

Contact between the adults using Shared Lives and children is often rare and most services would view it through the lens of risk. There are some people using Shared Lives who cannot safely have unsupervised contact with children, and they are matched accordingly, but the children of Shared Lives carers typically talk, not in terms of risk, nor even exclusively in terms of helping others, but also about the benefits they feel from their unusual lifestyle. Niamh says, "It has really shown me how lucky I am and not to take things for granted, it has made me appreciate what I have in my life when other people may be a bit less fortunate than me". She takes an instinctively asset-based approach to the people with whom she comes into contact, as aware of their capacity for fun as their needs:

The first time that I met Hilda she was a bit shy, but as she has grown to know me more she isn't as shy. Every time Hilda comes to our house she always makes me smile and laugh. She always has a smile on her face which makes everyone else smile.

As a care assistant in my 20s, I could have learned a lot from Niamh.

Nearly everyone using Shared Lives reports making and keeping friends and a third appear to make five or more new friends. Friendship is one of the most important aspects of most of our lives, but it cannot be bought or provided and brings risks, so it is another topic which most services skirt around. As a former Director of Adult Services puts it, "We offer people a service, but they are usually looking for a relationship". That combination of improved wellbeing, new relationships and achieving improved legal and financial status adds up to complete transformation for many: "[Shared Lives] has helped their journey from an inmate in a mental institution to a free, active and happy life. A person who now has a girlfriend, regular contact with his family and enjoys life as any senior citizen should – he is happy!" (Shared Lives Plus, 2015).

> One of my ladies was terrified to go outside. She can't read, write, tell the time and has no concept of time. She had never travelled alone. She now accesses the public bus service herself alone on foot, crosses busy roads, gets on the right bus and gets to college alone and returns alone. This lady is blind in one eye and has a cataract in the other. She has made lots of friends of her own. She has a voluntary role in a cafe taking money and orders as well as making food and clearing away. (Shared Lives Plus, 2015)

Those improvements in wellbeing are only now beginning to be captured systematically, through an academically produced measuring approach. Previously, like other 'community' services, Shared Lives providers had to rely on stories to evidence outcomes not considered important enough for the mainstream care system to invest in measuring. But those 'soft' outcomes resulting from forming caring and social relationships have turned out to be crucial to achieving the hard legal status of full citizen: Shared Lives carers described the battle required to help someone who had no birth certificate or other identification documents and who was no longer in touch with any living relatives to get a passport, or even just open a bank account. Without these keys, the door of citizenship and community would have always remained locked. With them, half of people within Shared Lives had gone on their first ever holiday, with half of those going abroad for the first time.

Each relationship is different, but the conditions for those relationships are deliberately constructed, following a shared national model. Two approaches in particular could be applied to a wide range of long-term support services:

- First, much more time and care is spent recruiting Shared Lives carers through an approval process which can take several months rather than several hours.
- Second, people who have been approved to take part are matched with people who need support. Both parties choose with whom they form a supportive relationship.

These two approaches in turn make possible different approaches to relationships and risk which can feel simple and human, rather than complex and stultifying.

Investing in finding the right people instead of replacing the wrong ones

Most long-term support services recruit people quickly and require them to work with whomever they are assigned to. The hidden costs of this in staff turnover and disciplinaries, described in Chapter Two, are enormous. Many front-line care workers and unqualified health workers are miraculously dedicated and conscientious despite the lack of respect, reward and care they receive from their employers (care workers in the UK have almost twice the national average suicide rate (CLG, 2017)), but a significant proportion of them are not, so time-consuming checking and monitoring systems leave as little room for human error as possible, councils spend large amounts trying to monitor their problematic contractors, and government spends nearly £200 million a year in England on inspectors to identify the frequent failures.

Shared Lives starts with a recruitment process that lasts at least three months. As well as the usual application form, references and interview, local coordinators will spend time getting to know the prospective Shared Lives carer, the home to which they intend to welcome people for support and the rest of their household who will need to feel comfortable with the idea of one, two or in some cases three extra members. This process is time-consuming, but essential if people are to spend extended periods with a disabled or older adult without direct supervision. Coordinators have to feel confident that the Shared Lives carer will stay within the broad terms of the role and the goals outlined in each individual's care plan, and will contact them if they are in difficulty or unsure of something. The approval process ends with a quality assurance panel in which existing Shared Lives carers, people who use Shared Lives and representatives of other Shared Lives schemes review the approval, in some cases talking with the applicant. The registered manager of each local scheme knows they will be held legally accountable for the safety and effectiveness of the care which takes place within each household for which they are responsible.

Few people would be willing to engage in a three-month recruitment process, if their reward at the end of it was an insecure, minimum wage, zero-hours contract to provide rushed, minimum standard care. The recruitment process is not only rigorous, it is also how the local coordinator builds a relationship with the Shared Lives carer and their family. Good schemes involve prospective participants in social activities with others who are further down the road. Those relationships not only create a deeper and more multifaceted picture of the participant, but ensure their mindset is in relational, not purely professional, mode.

Other models use the same principle of investing in recruiting the right people rather than managing the wrong ones, including the impressive Buurtzorg model in the Netherlands which I will return to later. The small-scale care and support microenterprises mentioned in Chapter Five also self-organise and rely on building relationships with local people who value and help shape their service, although they typically have to stay out of the realm of regulated care in order to do this lawfully and without incurring prohibitive regulatory costs.

The result of its different investment model is that Shared Lives costs on average £26,000 a year less for people with learning disabilities and £8,000 less for people with mental health problems (Todd and Williams, 2013) than comparable forms of regulated care. If all areas caught up with those using Shared Lives most, another 35,000 people would use it, immediately saving over £220 million (Shared Lives Plus, 2017). These would be largely real, cash savings, as the commissioner stopped paying for more expensive forms of care, rather than the 'savings' often attributed to new models which could only be realised were other services to be cut.

Offering a relationship not a service

One of the basic values of professional service delivery is impartiality. A professional has no favourites and maintains a detached relationship with her clients within clear professional boundaries. They avoid disclosing personal information about themselves and keep their lives inside and outside of work separate, avoiding socialising with their clients.

The need for boundaries of this kind is usually described as being for reasons which are therapeutic (the client needs clarity and for the worker to model 'appropriate' and non-exploitative relationships) and protective of the worker's health and reputation (if you spend time with clients outside of the professional environment, a client could make an allegation that was hard to disprove). There are some professions where there is a clear therapeutic theory behind this, notably counselling and psychotherapy, where the relationship is deliberately one in which the therapist is a 'blank sheet'.

But most public service roles are not following a therapeutic model of this kind. Policies and training manuals gloss over the real reason that support relationships need clear professional boundaries: not to be therapeutic, but because they mitigate the potentially harmful power imbalances that are inherent in traditional models of public service and the one-sided relationships within them. The worker necessarily learns intimate details of each client in assessing them, planning or delivering intimate or medical care. The client has a great deal invested in these relationships at a time when they may be lonely, frightened and desperate. Most professionals take their roles very seriously, but they have much less at stake. To invest emotionally in clients risks 'burn out'. These people are not their friends: they are a client, a customer, a case in their case load. People in health services are patients, or to senior managers, just 'beds'. (A manager in housing support services described to me the efforts their sector was making to talk about people and their homes, rather than units, stock and voids.) The current approach to forming support relationships is to bring together two people in crisis: the personal crisis of the support seeker and the ongoing professional crisis of the hard-pressed public service worker.

Impersonality protects each from the other's crisis. It also enables a simpler approach to referral and 'patient flow', as people are moved around the system like chess pieces. In contrast, professionals who begin to refer people to their local Shared Lives scheme often lose patience with finding that there is no 'match' for an individual who fits the referral criteria. For a system which is increasingly focused on short-term survival, taking time to match people can seem like a luxury, and the medium- to long-term benefits of a stable support relationship less compelling than a quick fix. Matching people would become much easier if it was a principle applied across all long-term support services, because the more people involved and looking for matches, the more compatible matches can be found.

The expectation of detachment sits uncomfortably with many working in front-line public services who were attracted to those professions because they have high levels empathy, compassion and emotional intelligence, as well their own needs, such as the need to help others, to make a difference, to be needed. Many people working in mental health services for instance, will have their own experience of mental distress.

Removing detached, professional boundaries from traditional public services would be disastrous. Within the current power imbalances, clients would be more likely to be exploited and professionals would burn out attempting to care more deeply for a succession of needy strangers. Detachment is the only manageable relationship one worker can have with numerous service users. But were we to reform our support services around bringing people together into more human relationships, more human approaches to boundaries would become possible.

There are boundaries within Shared Lives of course, but they are designed not around service users behaving 'appropriately' during a visit from a paid stranger, but to fit with life within a household which *both* parties have chosen to build. People living in Shared Lives households go on holiday together, are together at Christmas and other festivals and see each other happy, grumpy, tired, ill and overexcited. Both parties witness the intimacy of each other's close family relationships and talk of each other as 'just part of the family'.

The matching process is not complex: it begins with the local coordinator thinking about who might get on, based on shared hobbies, backgrounds or senses of humour. People then meet each other, spend increasing amounts of time together and discuss the possibility of a long-term match.

Matching is not just about whether the Shared Lives carer can meet the individual's needs. It is as much about whether they both feel like they will get on: do they 'click'? It is not just their relationship which is at stake: the Shared Lives carer has to be confident that their own partner, family and anyone else living in the household will similarly get on well with the individual. Love cannot be faked or simulated as part of a professional vocation. If the individual has a family of their own, there will often be a close bond between the two families: as one parent put it, "it's just like extending your own family". The mother of a young woman who moved in to Shared Lives at a point of family crisis said, "She started to talk about things with her brother and sister and realised from the beginning that her family could be part of her shared life – or not – if she so wished – it wasn't a case of one or the other."

Chris says,

> First I went to visit a Shared Lives carer twice but at that time he wasn't ready for a permanent arrangement. Then it was a visit to see if I liked [Alison], then a stop overnight. Then a final meeting to set up for moving. At first I walked the dog sometimes. I sorted out my bedroom, my bus pass, medication and medical treatment. I got to know the area and met Alison's family and friends.

I also stay with Sylvia and Carol for respite, they are Shared Lives carers too. I would say it is more of a family. I do get on with everybody – I get on very good with Pilui (Alison's husband), I get on with Alison very good, I would say more of a closeness.

One of the interesting features of matching is that the appearance of a match on paper is often trumped by the compatibility which only becomes apparent when people meet. It can be assumed for instance that people prefer to be matched within their culture or religion. One Shared Lives scheme matched a man recovering from stroke with a Shared Lives carer who spoke his community language, which was of particular benefit to his family who spoke little English. But another household has members of three separate world religions (the Shared Lives carer says every day is a festival).

Could other long-term support services match individuals with their workforce? Research in psychotherapy has found that the quality of relationship was the key factor in its impact, regardless of the support model used (Norcross, 2011). Many Direct Payment holders recruit their own staff, effectively matching themselves to their workers, with surveys consistently suggesting they are happier with their support than those using traditional models. However, there has been no cost comparison of matched and non-matched versions of traditional support services, to examine whether the greater investment needed to form such relationships was outweighed by savings from much reduced levels of failure and staff sickness and turnover, and the health gains of more effective relationships. And there is little possibility of mainstream services moving to a model of this kind until people buying services on behalf of the state start demanding better outcomes for their money, rather than lower unit costs.

Independence or interdependence?

During the 2000s, when tax receipts rose on the back of a growing economy and a Left-wing government increased public spending, the 'gold standard' of independent living was for many 'a flat of your own with your own front-door key'. Many people with a learning disability or mental health problem established tenancies with a rota of visiting staff. This model could be expensive for some, as the economies of scale of a large care home were replaced by one-to-one staff ratios, but for many people it was worth it: they achieved unheard of levels of independence. For others, independence was illusory. The services supporting them may have been called 'community' services, but their support was largely with practical skills: self-care, cooking and paying the bills, not with building relationships or being an active community member. The mother of a man with a significant mental health problem described to me how he had been moved from a group home where his health was stable, to a flat by himself, in the name of his own independence, despite neither he nor her thinking it was a good idea. "He hears the voices much more when he is on his own. And this wasn't a lovely flat in a lovely neighbourhood, it was on a sink estate. 'The community' were never going to be turning up on his doorstep bearing casseroles."

'Mate crime' sits alongside independent living like its cracked and distorted mirror. It refers to people befriending people with learning disabilities or mental health problems and exploiting or abusing them. This ranges from the depressing to the deadly. One group of young people with Asperger's talk about their 'Tuesday friends': a particular group of people who turn up and help them to the cashpoint on the day that their benefits get paid, then accompany them to the pub and help them spend all their money, disappearing until next benefits day.

People with learning disabilities experiencing mate crime are in a double-bind: considered too independent to be protected, but often unable to raise complaints and not taken seriously when they do:

> I used to live in my own flat but my neighbours
> would shout names, kick and punch me. In the end I
> left and for two years I slept rough. I'd only go home
> once a week for a shower. I didn't think much of the
> police – they didn't do their job. They didn't treat it
> seriously or even take a statement. (Walker, 2011b)

Another says:

> I moved out of a group home and for about a year
> I was living in my own place. But then a group of
> boys started causing trouble. They'd yell names, shout
> abuse and knock on windows. I couldn't relax and
> it went on for about a year. It made me nervous and
> depressed. The police tried to be helpful but they
> didn't do enough. It probably felt like an everyday
> thing to them. But it wasn't for me. In the end I had
> to give up my home. (Walker, 2011b)

Sometimes this escalates into much more serious crime:

> My brother was befriended by neighbours. They
> robbed him of several items and also stored drugs in
> his flat so that if the police raided their flat, nothing
> would be found. The police were generally very nice
> to him but were not happy about the drugs issue and
> said he should know it was wrong. My brother had
> never had friends before. (Autism Together, 2015)

Gemma Hayter was found dead on a disused railway embankment
in 2010. Two men and a woman were jailed for life for her
murder, with two others sentenced for manslaughter. She had
been forced to drink urine from a beer can, beaten with a mop
and stripped before being left for dead. Hayter had considered all
five to be her friends. A review found that none of the agencies
involved with her knew her relationship with the five killers,
but it was known that she was a regular victim of 'mate crime'.
The council's 'apology' was defensive:

> While the report has found that Gemma's murder
> could not have been prevented, we are sorry that
> Gemma did not receive more support to help her live
> a better life. We apologise sincerely for the failings
> identified in the report ... This complex case raises
> the challenge for all local authorities on how to
> safeguard vulnerable adults who have the right to

make their own decisions and may not always accept support. (Walker, 2011a)

Gemma Hayter is just one of the victims of a string of upsetting murders of people whose learning disabilities, mental ill health or other condition made them lonely and vulnerable: Susan Whiting was raped and murdered by a couple who befriended her and lured her to their house. Phillip Nicholson was lured to a flat in a Bournemouth by another couple who then stabbed him. 'Vulnerable adult' Jimmy Prout was tortured and murdered by five people he thought of as friends.

While the perpetrators are to blame for their crimes, not social workers, it is debatable that these crimes could not have been prevented, nor the victims enabled to live more safely, had they been supported to form positive relationships and efforts made to find allies in the community.

While the independence of some 'supported living' packages can turn out to be precarious if there is no plan or resources for supporting positive relationships, a supportive household can be a stable base for more sustainable independence. Clare moved in with her Shared Lives carers at a point when her own family was going through a difficult time. Her mum said in a letter to Clare's Shared Lives carers, 'The service provided a safe place. This became Clare's and the rest of the family's most used word in those early days. She talked openly about the trials and tribulations but feeling safe was the foundation.'

Clare says,

> Lots of people like me are just told about living in flats. My life was a disaster before I moved in [to Shared Lives]. It got better when I met [my Shared Lives carers]. I was a bit shy at first. It's hard to know what good is when you have not had it. More people need to know about Shared Lives. They need to know it is not about being stuck in a flat on your own. It is not about being lonely. It is about family. It is about having choices. It is just lovely. It is a good life. (Speech to Shared Lives Plus conference, 2015)

Shared Lives carer, Alison, says of Chris,

> He seems to feel a greater sense of freedom – he
> makes more choices, comes and goes as he pleases
> and stays at home alone for agreed periods of time.
> He seeks permission much less and more often tells
> me what he is going to do instead of asking. He is
> encouraged to make his own decisions even if I don't
> agree with them – this is much harder for me than
> it is for Chris! We have many conversations about
> honesty – Chris gets better at telling me the truth
> rather than just what he thinks I want to hear, and
> understanding that if I don't like it then that is my
> problem and not his!
>
> His social circle has expanded dramatically – he has
> met so many new people and is a valued member
> of our family and social group. He still enjoys close
> contact with staff and residents at his former home
> and has begun to meet new people independently
> of us.[1]

Taking the right risks

No form of support – indeed no contact between two human
beings – is without risks, but the autonomy afforded to Shared
Lives carers after they passed the approval process and have been
successfully matched, enables them to focus more on the risks
and risk-taking which matter most to the individual, rather than
those that preoccupy the managers of more traditional services.
They have explicit permission to pursue 'ordinary family life'
(and on occasion perhaps are more inclined to seek forgiveness
than permission). Alison again:

> Perhaps the thing that (wrongly) surprised me is just
> how much it means to Chris to have 'less forms to
> fill in'. Assessments and safeguards are still there but
> are much less intrusive into his everyday life and
> more proportional ... Yes, Chris needs support, but
> no, he does not need a risk assessment ... or signed

permission from me whenever he wishes to spend the evening in the pub.

Chris says,

> There are less forms to fill in. I am more independent. I go to more places than before, like we just went to Brighton – I couldn't do that before, there would be a lot more people involved and a lot of planning. Our trip to Rome would have taken much longer to plan for example how many staff and clients were going. In residential I couldn't go out to a club without having to do a risk assessment and care plan. Since I moved in I think we have been on 9 trips.

With a staff team and regular shift changes, a strict routine is often the way in which tasks such as medication are organised to minimise mistakes. For Chris, this meant:

> In residential I had to take my tablets exactly 8 am and 6 pm, here I can take them earlier or later if I want. My tablets have also been reduced. In residential I had to have my meals at set times – breakfast at 8 o'clock, tea at 5 o'clock with other residents. Here is different I can eat earlier or later.

Alison adds:

> Chris asks us things, tells us things, seeks advice, ignores advice, makes us laugh, infuriates us, socialises with us, spends time alone, cooks the dinner, refuses to cook the dinner and has good days, bad days and days in between. Normal family life … And from this stems from greater freedom underpinned by a greater sense of belonging. If and when he moves on for whatever reason then he will go with our blessing, but for the time being he is one of our family, this is his home and this is where he belongs.

Although inspectors' data[2] suggests that incidents are far rarer compared to all other forms of care, it would be wrong to pretend that Shared Lives is immune to mistakes, failures or even abuse.

There are some risks which come with the messiness of family life: Shared Lives carers who are a couple get divorced, for instance, or become too ill to carry on with their role. While there may be other family members who have been trained to step in temporarily at short notice, the model is designed around Shared Lives carers not being readily replaceable. The liminal position of a Shared Lives household: outside of a recognisable service domain, but not quite a 'normal' family, results in confusion around some kinds of 'incident' which would be considered entirely normal within a family, but a disciplinary matter within a staff team. For instance, when a Shared Lives carer and their partner have a row which is witnessed by the individual living with them, local scheme coordinators can wonder which frame of reference they should be using. This is particularly difficult if someone, such as a day-centre worker, reports their concern as a safeguarding incident. Once that process has been triggered, it can be very difficult for the professionals involved to exercise their judgement before a series of actions have been taken: usually starting with the immediate action of removing the individual from their home (in theory this requires a court order but the law is not always followed), then, conversely a seemingly endless process of investigating what actually happened. The system deals swiftly with the risks it can comprehend – a worker has abused a client – but is impervious to those it cannot: the risk that a person's household might be irrevocably damaged.

It is not that the risk of witnessing or even being on the receiving end of angry or even violent behaviour is entirely controlled within a traditional service, where an individual may regularly be affected by the behaviour of other service users. Chris says, "In Shared Lives it is a lot easier to get on with people – in residential you have to be careful what you say in case people take it the wrong way or someone kicks off." This is seen as an inevitable feature of services, not an infringement of Chris' rights, regardless of how much or little choice Chris had about who to live with.

By witnessing other's imperfect behaviour and what they do to rectify their mistakes, we can learn about how people try to form and repair relationships. This kind of learning is absent from the traditional service with its focus on behaviour which is 'appropriate' to a workplace, and 'inappropriate' behaviour seen as a professional 'challenge' to 'de-escalate'. But it takes a brave Shared Lives service manager to see the messiness of family life as a positive learning experience, knowing they will have to account for their pragmatism if something more serious is later found to have happened.

In one incident, a man with a learning disability who has limited communication skills was at his regular day service talking to a new member of staff, as his usual key worker was off sick. The staff member was shocked to hear the man describe an incident of violence and immediately raised a safeguarding alert. The man did not go home that evening, but instead was taken to a care home by social workers. In keeping with typical safeguarding procedures, the Shared Lives carers were not informed of the nature of the allegation pending an investigation. The next day, the key worker was back from sick leave and immediately identified that the man had, as he always did, been describing the previous night's episode of his favourite soap opera, which often featured people rowing and hitting each other. The man was returned to his home and household, but only after considerable distress for all concerned, which put the most important relationships in his life under unnecessary stress. He had also had his human rights unlawfully infringed by his summary removal from what had become his family home, by social workers acting outside of their legal powers. Had he been living in a more formal service, the service manager would probably have been contacted and a peer–to–peer discussion between the professionals would very likely have established the truth, but Shared Lives carers as self-employed people in an unfamiliar and unusual model fell between two stools with neither the status and respect of being regarded as professional colleagues nor recognition of the legal status of a family home.

Shared Lives carers, like home-care workers, work without direct supervision, but the levels of poor care within home care are much higher, according to CQC (CQC, 2017). The months-long selection and matching processes within Shared Lives probably account for a great deal of this difference. Many people receiving home care are also isolated and report seeing no one regularly other than the workers who visit them. Shared Lives carers are expected to help the individual who lives with them develop new friendships within the community. Being a visible member of our community, with a number of friendships and acquaintances, can keep us safe from the dangers of both isolation and of exploitation by people masquerading as friends.

The risk management approach could be described as more diffuse than a traditional service, where one disinterested or malign individual can influence the rest of a team, or poison the culture within a building, which then affects everyone living in that building. So in the Winterbourne View residential medical unit for people with learning disabilities, a whole team appears to have gone 'rotten'. In hospitals, poor management, leading to poor recruitment, induction and supervision can mean hundreds of deaths, as happened in the Mid Staffordshire Hospital. The usual mantra following such disasters is that 'lessons have been learned', but the lessons do not extend to the dangers inherent in operating on a large scale.

I am aware of one accusation of serious abuse at present in Shared Lives the UK and realistically, there must be others that have been undetected. These will have affected one or two people within that household, rather than the dozens or hundreds of the scandals mentioned earlier, but they will be horrific for the people involved and the relative safety of Shared Lives cannot be taken for granted. It is possible that, without the comfort of an ever-present manager, tightly prescribed roles and a high level of recording, Shared Lives staff teams have by necessity had to develop more relational approaches. One Shared Lives carer told me, "you feel personally accountable" rather than a cog in somebody else's system.

The expectation, even built into Shared Lives inspections, of living 'ordinary family life' is a powerfully straightforward ethos by which what is OK and what is not is judged, largely free of the enforced suspension of disbelief and cognitive dissonance that is required to maintain the idea of a service as a 'community setting'. As one Shared Lives carer who is also a registered nurse put it, "I'm using the same caring skills, but there are not the same power structures in my kitchen as there are in the hospital." Another says,

> in the care home the older person who lived with me had to wait until 6 pm for her painkillers no matter how bad her pain was. Fear of doing something wrong takes over common sense and it becomes about protecting the service or the staff not the person. In my house, she could have it when she needed it – she never asked to take more than the right dose. (Shared Lives carer)

It is hard to think of a more effective approach to reducing endemic failure within many of our services than rebalancing the power relationships within them and taking a clearer view of those imbalances that remain.

To see more territory returned to the community from its professional occupiers, we will need to establish a more stable, balanced set of expectations around risk and safety than the current wildly swinging pendulum within whose arc any service attempting to draw on normal life must currently operate.

Viewed from the perspective of people living in Shared Lives households, the greatest risk to their wellbeing may be the pressure that the model is constantly under to conform to traditional ideas, including that people should always move on from a 'service' before they develop 'dependence'. Shared Lives managers are often under pressure to see their Shared Lives carers as a resource to be exploited rather than sustained. In one or two areas Shared Lives carers have been treated like gig-economy employees (more managed, less trusted, expected to work with whomever the service decides and so on) without any employee benefits (such as hourly pay and sick pay). In these areas, Shared Lives carers have started to challenge their employment status, but it's a lose/lose situation: Shared Lives would neither work nor be affordable if people became employees of a traditionally managed service and its uniquely genuine, reciprocal relationships would founder.

Simple solutions to complex needs

Were Shared Lives only being used with a small number of people, or only with one group, it would be reasonable to be extremely sceptical of both its potential and the transferability of its approaches and ethos. The number of people using Shared Lives remains relatively small in comparison to around 500,000 living in care homes, but, despite modest investment and the public being largely oblivious, it has reached nearly 14,000 by 2017 through growth of up to 1,000 a year, at a time when all other forms of support are in retreat. People with learning disabilities remain the biggest group using Shared Lives, but it has been used successfully with an extremely diverse group of adults, including people with mental health problems, older people with dementia (who tend to visit their Shared Lives carer for short breaks and as an alternative to a day centre, rather than move in), people who need support to return home from hospital, young disabled people in transition to adulthood, care leavers, people at the end of life, ex-offenders, people who misuse substances and survivors of domestic violence. In each case, Shared Lives remains a simple combination of ordinary people with the capacity to care and a spare room, with a local organisation that can bring the right people together and monitor the results, but there are numerous examples of people thriving in Shared Lives who were found 'challenging' by the most expensive, highly staffed health, care and even criminal justice services.

This shows up in remarkable health outcomes for people previously extremely poorly served by the NHS. Many of these people have physical or learning disabilities, alongside physical health problems. A rapidly increasing proportion of NHS resources is taken up with people with two or more long-term conditions and it is these people for whom our single condition-focused NHS is most poorly designed. The health gains of the most 'complex' people who use Shared Lives, often achieved through the interventions of people with no formal health training, demonstrate that multiple needs do not have to be the NHS-crushing problem that they are at present. The same is true of most public services: there are few people in prison who do not have a mental health problem, a learning disability or a substance misuse problem and many have all three. Many homelessness services expect people to have addressed their alcohol or drug problems before they can be rehoused, but many alcohol and drug services are inaccessible to the homeless, or regard a settled base as necessary for therapeutic work to begin. Where people have support needs that stretch across several different conditions, there is often little communication, let alone cooperation, between the services they use. I remember vividly the account given by a wheelchair user with an alcohol problem who had been homeless. He was admitted to hospital and discharged – in his wheelchair – onto the street at the end of his treatment in the middle of winter. A couple of days later he was readmitted with life-threatening hypothermia.

Sharon has a lot of skills and can appear to be very capable, but was referred to a Shared Lives scheme during a personal crisis. She moved in with the Shared Lives carer in November. The scheme coordinator felt that if she stuck it out to the New Year that would be a success. Six months later, Sharon felt settled and that she was building towards getting her own place again at a manageable pace. A close relationship with a single Shared Lives carer had led to multiple improvements across many service boundaries:

> My depression has gone.
> I have stopped smoking.
> I am going to the gym 5 times a week.
> I am eating healthily.
> I have reduced my medication massively (soon to come off my last tablet).
> I am starting to build a relationship with my family.
> I am more happier in myself.
> My relationship with my boyfriend is getting better.
> I am learning to cook and bake.

The greater insight afforded by a deeper relationship can lead to better outcomes from other services:

They thought she was deaf until I investigated further and found she hadn't had her ears syringed for over five years. Easily sorted out by visit to Practice nurse at GP and her hearing is fine now. (Shared Lives Plus, 2015)

[He] was in a wheelchair due to being over-medicated, because his doctors thought he was very severely epileptic. We found out that most of his 'seizures' were behavioural, and they gradually reduced his epilepsy meds. From having around 4 'seizures' per day, he hasn't had any for 12 months. He now walks and attends college. The GP stated that this was directly attributable to care we had put in place. (Shared Lives Plus, 2015)

Darren, who has a learning disability, moved in with Shared Lives carers June and Rob when he was 18. He had been in a specialist foster care placement for offenders, having committed serious sexual offences within his own family, which had led to his being completed rejected by them. Due to the nature of his offences, he had to leave his foster placement at the age of 18. Because of the level of risk, probation and social services could find only one service willing to support him, in a secure facility costing £5,000 per week. June says,

We felt this lad wasn't been given any chance. I had worked as a mental health nurse working with people who had been sexually abused, so I was aware of the issues. We had a fantastic probation officer who saw him twice a week and a policeman who carried out risk assessments and talked bluntly about repercussions to Darren. Both were really helpful, as was the Shared Lives scheme worker.

However, the placement was not straightforward. As June recounts:

My husband and I were working in shifts to ensure that Darren never went more than 10 minutes unsupervised. That meant he could, for instance, go to the shop and back, provided he took less than 10 minutes. He could have no unsupervised contact with under 16s, so almost all activities were difficult to manage, but we tried to fit in lots of positive activities and trips – we didn't want to be constantly be on his back. We didn't take any breaks for two or three years because we couldn't find appropriate available accommodation. There had been an incident during one respite break, which meant we came home to a crisis.

Nevertheless the arrangement worked out. June again:

Darren has had lots of therapeutic work from professionals which we have reinforced and there has been no re-offending in six years. He works in a charity shop three days a week and plays football in a local club. These kinds of activities are easier to arrange now that he is a little older, because we can find activities with no under 18s involved. He is aiming to live in semi-independent accommodation.

Darren is very smiley and very vulnerable and lonely. He is desperate for friendship and can be taken for a ride. He is also a lot of fun and has a good sense of humour. He enjoys reading and watching Arsenal. He says if he hadn't come to us, he would be in prison.

An interesting detail of Darren and June's story is that, while they spent more than two years waiting for a break, because no service could be found which was willing to manage the risks associated with Darren's history, he now takes his breaks with June's grown-up son, who has no social care qualifications or experience, but who got to know Darren and form a bond with him over several years. When I heard that no break had been offered to June and her partner for more than two years I was astonished and angry: June's dedication was saving local services nearly a quarter of a million pounds a year; surely for a fraction of that they could have made safe arrangements.

Even more astonishing then, that something unachievable for any of the local services, even the most expensive and highly staffed, turned out to be achievable for a young man with no health or care background, at little or no cost. There will be some reading this who conclude that an unacceptable risk must have been taken, by placing such a high-risk individual with an unqualified breaks provider. But the real lesson is the limitations of what can be achieved by traditional services, no matter how well-resourced, and the potential for a relational approach to work even in these extreme circumstances.

Some of the most interesting applications of Shared Lives are in sectors where it is most countercultural. Shared Lives is being developed as a mental health service, including one NHS Trust which uses a very similar model to provide an acute mental health service, in which people either get out of a hospital ward, or avoid being admitted, through being matched with specially trained family hosts for a few weeks of intensive support in the hosts' household. I recall visiting a friend who had been admitted to a mental health ward housed in a Victorian hospital. It was hard to see anything uplifting or therapeutic in the ward environment, which was one in which most of us would feel dislocated, lacking in privacy and ill at ease. Receiving the same medical and psychological interventions while living in an ordinary family home, with people we have chosen to be with, would be preferable for many. One young woman living with a Shared Lives carer following a period in which she became very unwell with a long-term mental illness, felt that the family dog, which from early in her stay she was asked to take responsibility for walking at least once a day, was the single most beneficial intervention during that period.

Services designed to respond to a single issue affecting a single person not only struggle to respond to individuals with more than one issue, but also to the interlocking challenges faced by people within their families and relationships. Estimates of the number of parents with learning disabilities vary wildly from 23,000 to 250,000, partly because there are different definitions of 'learning disability', but there is consensus that the number is growing (WPTN, 2016). Similarly, estimates vary, but there are certainly thousands of parents with a mental health problem and there are large numbers of parents who have substance misuse problems and many more within abusive or violent relationships. Many are affected by two or more of these factors, but parenting support is not the focus or expertise of many of the relevant services, so parents facing multiple challenges tend to 'bounce off' various single-issue services, until, at crisis point, numerous services pile in.

For some parents who have learning disabilities (often along with other challenges), it is neither safe nor sensible to work towards the child remaining with the parents. But often multiple crisis responses are uncoordinated and entirely focused on the presenting risks with no ability to see, let alone build on, the potential capabilities of the parents. Before any accessible parenting support is offered, a child whose parents have mild learning disabilities is often within a court system, which sees the risks of the child remaining with its parents very clearly, but does not have to consider the risks of removing them (children in care have significantly lower rates of qualifications and higher rates of offending and poor mental health), and which may not be aware of available parenting support or in an area where budget cuts have ensured that there are none. A single residential parenting assessment costs up to £127,000, but only a third of assessed parents retain custody of their children (Munro et al, 2014).

We all find becoming a new parent challenging, but many of us have good incomes, support networks, access to good maternity and health services, the assertiveness skills to argue for what we need, and access to peer-support groups. Parents who have learning disabilities often have very low incomes, troubled or non-existent relationships with family (some of whom may feel strongly that they should not be in sexual relationships, let alone having children) and no peer-support network. They find manuals incomprehensible and the health service opaque. Any services they access may start from the viewpoint that they should not be having children and are unlikely to be able to parent.

The system takes their challenges and adds more as it examines every aspect of their lives for risk with a forensic approach under which nearly all of us would be found wanting in some respect. Some parents are assessed in specialist residential units, where they will know no one, be dislocated from their familiar surroundings and routines and far from home. This problem and risk-focused approach sets these parents up to fail. One parent recounts: "Everyone told me different things I had to do and I got very confused. I was so nervous about doing the right thing and worried about the baby being taken away and it just made me worse."

In May 2011, when she was 21, Lisa, who has a mild learning disability and hearing loss, found out she was pregnant. She had been taken away from her own family when she was 11 and put into foster care, and was now afraid that she might lose her home and that her baby would be taken away from her. She couldn't cook, use a washing machine or manage money and was struggling living on her own. Lisa is one of the few parents with learning disabilities who have been offered the chance to live with a Shared Lives carer, in a household that recreates the natural support of an older, experience parent or grandparent. Shared Lives South West arranged for Lisa to live with Dawn (and her husband and two sons) for six months. Lisa then moved to her own two-bedroom flat with her six-month-old baby, with regular visits from Dawn (Greenstreet, 2011).

Could we apply this ethos to all public services?

The practices and principles at the heart of Shared Lives are rarely applied to other public services. It is, however, part of a family of approaches that between them work with thousands of people.

One with a close similarity to Shared Lives is Homeshare, in which an older person who has low-level support needs or has become isolated, and who has a spare room, is matched with (usually) a younger person who needs somewhere to live. The younger person does not pay rent for their room but helps out and provides companionship. The older person is also often providing a young person with a start in life and both reduce the risk of loneliness which can affect people of all ages. This model is used by several hundred older people across the UK through over 20 local schemes, but is much more significant in other countries and there is an international movement of organisations collectively supporting thousands. Homeshare is used by people who have low-level support needs and do not need intimate, personal care, so its processes are lighter touch, but it also involves a matching process, in which people decide with whom to share their homes. It enables both parties to meet their different needs and to contribute to each other's welfare in a reciprocal relationship. It has the potential to be a way for tens of thousands of older people who do not want to 'downsize' to use their unused spare rooms. Older people say they value giving a younger person (who may also be isolated having moved to a new city for work or study) a good home and a start in life, as much as they value the help and companionship. There is no reason Homeshare could not grow to the scale of mainstream housesharing concepts such as the globally successful Airbnb.

Circles of support, such as those developed by the PLAN organisation in Canada or more recently by Community Circles in the UK, are often built around an individual who has a learning disability or other lifelong impairment. Family, friends and supporters are connected into an evolving but lifelong supportive network which advocates for the individual, supports coordination of their care and maintains social connections. PLAN founder Vickie Cammack developed an application called Tyze which used social media technology to help circles to form, stay connected and active. Community Circles has developed the model for use by older people in care homes among a wide range of other groups. For 25 years, KeyRing supported living networks have used a circles approach, in which a group of people with learning disabilities or other support needs are connected socially to each other to help each other out and meet up regularly, with either a community-living volunteer or another form of support who is provided with housing to live locally, to provide practical help with things like reading bills and to meet up and explore their neighbourhood.

Intentional communities such as the Camphill communities or L'Arche involve disabled and non-disabled people, or other mutually supportive groups, living communally, often with a shared religious faith or another strong mutual bond. Participants either live in a linked group of properties owned by the group, or in a large shared house.

Earlier I looked at the hundreds of small community enterprises that are built from small groups of people finding shared goals and often sharing their resources and creativity. Later I'll discuss Local Area Coordination, in which neighbourhood-based coordinators have the time and space to form relationships with isolated or vulnerable people and to reconnect them with their communities.

It is in the interests of our established care and health industries to dismiss all of these initiatives as either small-scale or untested, but what would happen if, instead, we reshaped those public services that need a long-term relationship with people, around those relationships? The next chapter sets out how a rehumanised model of long-term support could be built around the lessons from Shared Lives and allied approaches. This would not just be a model for early or 'preventative' interventions, but could be applied to every service that needs to have more than a brief relationship with an individual or family.

Almost everything about our public services would change:

- Instead of managing employee turnover and failure we would invest in giving the right people (including people who need support themselves) as much responsibility, access to resources and autonomy as possible.
- People and worker(s) would choose each other and form lasting support relationships.
- We would use more ordinary homes and spare rooms and fewer service buildings.
- More would consistently be expected of us in relation to our own wellbeing and that of those close to us, but we would be able to access more training, expertise and backup in return.
- Our services would value our wellbeing, independence, social connections and resilience as much as the mitigation or management of our symptoms or problems.

To do this, we would have to be willing to recognise and then finally dismantle the invisible asylums that, despite our best instincts, we repair and rebuild every day.

Escaping the invisible asylum: actions

1. Recruit the right people, rather than managing the wrong ones

A key lesson from Shared Lives is that you can give people a great deal of autonomy in long-term support roles, which enables them to provide better support while enjoying their job more, providing you invest in really careful recruitment. Currently many support workers are recruited as quickly and cheaply as possible, while medical practitioners are recruited for technical competence, but with less attention paid to whether they can listen, communicate and empathise in order to use that competence effectively.

2. Aim for real relationships

People will move heaven and earth for people they have come to regard as friends or family, not as 'customers' or 'clients'. This only happens when both individual and worker can choose each other. This matching process, following careful recruitment, could be applied to almost any long-term support service.

3. Aim for wellbeing and resilience

Whatever else is going on in someone's life, they are likely to dream of living a good life in a good place, with something meaningful to do and people to love. Services that pay these overarching personal goals no mind, but focus exclusively on a single problem or need, are unlikely to succeed.

SEVEN

Designing a new national health and wellbeing service

'Sarah' had a lifetime of severe mental distress, rejection and addiction problems before she was supported to live independently, funded through a personal budget. Despite having a diagnosis of schizophrenia, Sarah had often been unable to access local inpatient mental health services because of bed shortages and had spent time in prison and residential care. In May 2010 Sarah took on a supported tenancy for a two-bedroom flat provided by the Amber Trust. She had very little self-esteem and confidence so she was offered the opportunity to become involved in the Trust's allotment project. Initially very anxious, Sarah's confidence grew so she could make her own way to the allotment with the friends she had made there, and after two years, become a volunteer 'buddy' to support newcomers to the project. Her confidence and independence grew so much that she is moving on from supported accommodation to a home where she will have her own tenancy.

(Bennett, 2014)

There are many critiques of health and care services, but few that go on to describe an affordable, politically achievable alternative, partly because, as Shared Lives and the related models described in Chapter Six remain under-researched and easy to overlook, no such model was seen to provide a substantial enough evidence base. That evidence trap remains and many will dwell on the risks of rapidly adopting practices that have not been thoroughly researched. Meanwhile the risks of continuing with the same model manifest themselves in increasingly bleak realities.

In this chapter I will outline the transition I think we need to make and the long-term support system that will result from making it: what kinds of interventions and relationships it will create and contain; how it will be resourced (not just with money but also with time and creativity from those currently seen as recipients or customers), what it will value and what its rules and expectations will be.

Wellbeing: aligning public services around a single goal

It is astonishing that, despite constant talk of 'integrating' health and social care, you will never hear anyone suggest that health and care, much less other public services, should share a unified goal. How services could become 'integrated' when they have different goals and pay provider organisations for different things escapes me. There is not even a sense of a single goal or set of goals within the NHS, much less between health, care, housing, criminal justice and other long-term support services.

For a coherent new public service system, we will need a single goal; one not just be expressed in strategy documents but also in payment systems, inspection and performance management.

In the final report of their Connected Communities partnership, the RSA defines wellbeing as

> a key social value that can be generated by a socially productive (as opposed to merely financially efficient) approach to public policy, representing as it does the satisfaction that citizens have with their lives, the relative amounts of suffering or comfort they experience, and the realisation of their potential and aspirations. (Parsfield et al, 2015: 11)

The *Care Act 2014* sets achieving and maintaining wellbeing as the overarching goal for social care, defining it broadly to include physical and mental health, housing, meaningful activity (employment or volunteering), positive family life and dignity.

These are not goals that services can achieve alone; they are goals we and our families can only achieve for ourselves, with the right help. A system that is set up to maximise wellbeing cannot wait for crises, which often leave unrepairable damage (the older person who never regains mobility after a fall; the parent with a mental health problem who loses custody of their child). It must act early and consistently, building resilience and connection through every intervention.

As an overarching goal for all public services, wellbeing would realign services' goals with our goals and would drive behaviour changes in two crucial ways. First, it is intrinsically empowering. We cannot experience wellbeing if we are powerless, dependent and unable to contribute. Second, wellbeing is something we experience mainly through our relationships with other people. Our relationships with people paid to support us are important in this, but much more important are our relationships with our friends, family and neighbours. Few of us can achieve a good life in isolation – and isolation and loneliness are the biggest threats to wellbeing for millions of older, disabled and mentally ill people – so a wellbeing-based system must be able to interact constructively with households, families and communities as well as with individuals.

Wellbeing is set down in legislation as social care's goal but that is not reflected in the *economics* of social care, which are dominated by payments for time spent carrying out physical care tasks for people. Social care services are not paid more to help people become more independent of support; achieving this leads to a *loss* of income as the individual requires less worker time. Services cannot get paid for supporting families who care for one of their members to become more self-supporting units, with the tailored range of care, advice, training and backup interventions that would require. The NHS's five-year strategy has a chapter on community and people power, but again, those concepts are absent from NHS economics: the hospital tariff system rewards activity rather than outcome. If a hospital and its local partners reduced the need for hospital treatments, the hospital would probably go bust. If the hospital becomes more efficient and treats more people, its commissioners go bust.

Despite the misalignment between ideas of wellbeing and the short termism of current public service economics, many professionals already think holistically and beyond their job roles, despite the professional risks of so doing. Adopting a single shared goal would liberate all public service workers to do the same. Hazel Stuteley and her colleague were struggling to achieve public health gains as a health visitor on a deprived estate in Cornwall. Stepping outside of their roles, they convened a community group, which began with five residents who each had challenges of their own: "They didn't look like a group that was going to change the world." That group became the Beacon Project which went on to transform life for hundreds of people, managing a £2.2 million budget, with outcomes as diverse as postnatal depression rates down by 77%, and crime down by 50% (Chanan, 2011). Refocusing on good lives in a good place freed professionals from narrow job roles, but enabled them to achieve real health outcomes.

There may seem something perverse in suggesting that the way to personalise public services around people's deeply individual needs is to set those services a single, one-size-fits-all goal. Wellbeing of course is a set of linked goals, which gives it breadth and flexibility (one of the risks of adopting it would be that different service sectors would try to redivide themselves to pursue only 'their' part of the overarching agenda). But, while it collects several goals together, wellbeing is also a simple enough conceptual framework to capture the idea of living a good life in terms we can all understand, without falling back on outcomes which are directed only at disabled or older people (Halpern, 2010). Government already tracks the whole population's wellbeing via a series of survey questions about happiness, anxiety, a sense of purpose and so on. The Young Foundation developed a wellbeing and resilience measurement that was used with whole neighbourhoods in cities across Europe (Cooke and Muir, 2012). A major programme of research called *Realising the Value of People and Communities* (Wood, Finnis, Khan and Ejbye, 2016) identified the real economic value of taking a wellbeing and community-orientated approach.

From that set of broad goals would need to be developed a single set of aims, outcome measures, a single performance management system and one approach to paying for what works and penalising what does not. This chapter attempts to set out what those would look like.

Three key tests for future public services: are they asset-based, future-focused and do they connect people?

Earlier, I drew attention to two key aspects of the concept of wellbeing that make it a strong candidate for being the overarching goal of a wide range of public services: that it is intrinsically empowering and that it is relational. I also suggested that wellbeing as a goal, in place of more medical or narrowly framed goals, would, if built into performance and payment systems, push public services towards acting preventatively as well as reactively. The cultures and behaviours of these new public services would look very different to those we see today, with services needing to pass three new tests.

Test One: is every intervention asset-based?

> I shouldn't have to spend my life proving that my son can't do things, to get the support my family needs to help him do things for himself.

This quotation from an unpaid family carer illustrates the catch-22 situation that people accessing services face; social care is supposed to help people to achieve wellbeing and the NHS to achieve good health, but the fences and gates we construct and maintain around services requires people to subjugate themselves to a dehumanised bureaucracy before accessing help. The means test involves demonstrating a degree of poverty. The eligibility test involves highlighting people's needs and minimising their strengths, skills and informal support networks. Once inside the gates, services fear relinquishing control over the risks in people's lives and letting go of the person. Should the individual give up the support they have accessed, they risk never regaining it.

Kretzmann and McKnight (1993) and others developed the concept of asset-based thinking from their observations of the ways in which people or even whole communities were labelled as broken, failing or deficient. In response, a range of services would attempt to do things for people that they had previously done for themselves. The attempt to help was well-intentioned but as people become less confident of their own capacity to care for and help others without professional input, so we become, in McKnight's phrase, a *Careless Society* (McKnight, 1995), locked into co-dependency with the growing number of people who rely for their livelihoods on supporting us.

An asset-based approach starts not with the question, 'Which of our services do you want?' but, 'What does a good life look like to you and how can we work together to achieve it?' It is to look first for what an individual, family or community can do or could do with help, rather than only at what they cannot do right now. These questions can ultimately only be answered by people themselves, because a good life looks different to each of us. The role of the supporter is to get to know the individual, to understand and help them to understand their capacity and to work with them to build their capacity, confidence and resilience. It is not just those with low-level support needs who have capacity and assets: everyone has capacity and the potential to build it.

The Blair/Brown Labour government (1997-2010) invested in public services. NHS waiting times and mortality rates reduced: a significant achievement. But the overall health of the nation did not increase. In fact, people's lifestyles, including diets and levels of exercise, became less healthy. Lifespans increased faster than *healthy* lifespans. This was not some perverse result of improving healthcare, but improving healthcare did not address those health and wellbeing factors; nor could they. There was investment in public health initiatives, but the dominant model of experts telling people what was healthy failed to engage with what motivates us to keep ourselves and those we love well.

Blunt instruments such as increased taxes and laws banning smoking in public spaces show some evidence of being effective, but cannot be applied to all areas of life: calories are hard to ban or tax; no democracy could force sedentary people to take exercise and you cannot pass a law against loneliness. Some aspects of health and wellbeing – teenage pregnancy, most kinds of crime – improved rapidly under Labour, but the reasons for changes of this kind often cannot always be reliably and solely traced back to any policy or service initiative; they are equally likely to be about cultural and demographic changes. At present, for instance, mental distress is rising among teenage girls, but falling among boys, while risky behaviours associated with poor mental health are falling for both groups (Lessof et al, 2016).

During the boom years many councils increased and improved their services and introduced 'customer service' culture into their dealings with the public. But their 'customers' developed commensurately high expectations, and some felt their own responsibility was simply to pay their taxes, choose between options and complain when things went wrong.

During an unusually cold winter some years ago, an elderly couple died, apparently of cold and neglect. They did not have family or friends nearby to help them stay warm, fed and well, as heavy snow kept them housebound. It was clear that people did care: neighbours reported trying repeatedly to persuade the local council to respond to their concerns. It was striking though that, while they had spent considerable amounts of time and energy in trying to get a service from the council, they had not apparently thought to use that time to support their neighbours themselves. The elderly couple could have been helped by a range of services, but arguably, hot food, an invitation to a warm house, help with shopping and so on are not intrinsically professional services; they could equally have been offered by any member of the community. Perhaps the neighbours involved not only felt that it was the council's responsibility, not theirs, to help frail older people, but also that they would have been doing something questionable and open to misinterpretation if they had 'interfered'.

Taken to its logical extreme, the asset-based critique of public services could see all support services as liable to crowd out personal, family and community action and do more harm than good. McKnight was not arguing for this, but he did argue to remove power (particularly monopolies over areas of community life and wellbeing) and money from state agencies. He suggested placing power directly in the hands of individuals (through personal budgets) and communities (through community development work). This book draws on asset-based thinking, but I do not believe that the activities of citizens and of the state are necessarily in opposition.

A lesson of the success of the Shared Lives movement is that state resources and infrastructure are needed. Shared Lives is regulated and inspected; it is funded largely with state money; it has local organisations to coordinate it and a national infrastructure and community of practice. But infrastructure can be used sparingly to avoid smothering the individual strength of individuals, families and communities with blanket approaches.

Even emergency and crisis interventions can see the whole person and build on their assets. Failing to do so means taking big decisions about a person's life (Where will this older person live on leaving hospital? Can this parent in a mental health crisis parent their child safely?) during or in the immediate aftermath of a crisis (a fall and broken hip; a psychotic episode), when it is hardest to see the capacity and potential of the individual and their struggling support networks. In the aftermath of a crisis, seeing clearly what is broken and the risks, but lacking an in-depth knowledge of the person's life, it is easy to assume that what is broken is broken permanently, or can only be fixed with extended professional input. An asset-based approach by crisis services would see them invest more of their scarce time in talking with the individual and those close to them. They would see their vital work in a wider context. Rather than looking with despair on the rising tide of crises flooding towards them and trying to build their admission boundaries higher, they would make themselves more easily available in small doses to back up community services and families, reducing the pressure and anxiety in those systems.

Unrealistic beliefs about the value of the service's own assets are wrapped up in the deficit-focused approach many services take to people. As noted earlier, the service sees only the potential benefits of its own support and expertise, ignoring the potential harm that being removed from their natural ecosystem can do to an individual. Individuals working within these services often have an acute awareness of the gap between their employer's rhetoric and what they can realistically help someone achieve, which they experience as professional guilt, cynicism and, in some cases, 'burn out'.

This is not to devalue our public services, whose professionals cannot work miracles. A system is only asset-based if it recognises the value and potential of every element of the system, including state services and the humans who work within them. Neither does an asset-based system ignore the needs and problems of either individuals or of services; it takes a realistically optimistic view of both.

Asset-based approaches find it difficult to thrive within a wider system which is deficit-focused or is in constant crisis mode. They value different things and work on different timescales. Asset-based approaches that rely on building mutual understanding and trust are fatally undermined if the individual runs up against a part of the system that can only see them as a risk, cost or problem. So, it is only possible to introduce asset-based thinking effectively if it is applied system-wide, under the banner of the single wellbeing goal. This would need to be accompanied by a single approach to first contact, planning and assessment, in place of the multiple assessments people endure as they meet multiple services.

Making access to support easier is often dismissed as 'opening the floodgates'. At present, desperate or damaged people may attempt to access numerous 'inappropriate' crisis services, each of which will separately try to screen them out at great time and expense. An asset-based approach takes a counter-intuitive approach to reducing demand on services, through offering earlier support to more people, but focusing that early support, and each subsequent intervention, primarily on helping people to build their own confidence, expertise, connections and resilience. This would replace our 'all or nothing' approach with moving more people into lower levels of support while reducing the number in crisis. People with long-term support needs, who believe that expert support will be readily available when needed, are more likely to feel confident in choosing lower levels of support (with the commensurate reduction in intrusion into their lives), when they can. We could all call on emergency services constantly, but we don't. Where people started to draw on expensive support services unnecessarily, a community-based intervention like Local Area Coordination can help people develop their capacity to stay well, addressing the reasons behind their behaviour.

Asset-based thinking cannot only be applied at the level of the individual: if we believe that people are experts in what works for them, it follows that that expertise should also inform service and system planning: the practice of 'co-production', discussed later, describes how this can happen. The introduction of personal budgets suffered from not drawing on this expertise: because their insights are lacking from service planning, many personal-budget holders find only the same old familiar services are on offer rather than genuinely new choices.

A disabled-people-led human rights organisation called CHANGE has demonstrated how people with learning disabilities, typically assumed to be unable to work or to be employable only in the most menial jobs, can take on leadership roles. CHANGE uses a co-worker model, in which an individual with a learning disability is employed to share a role with a non-disabled colleague, both paid equally. They combine their respective strengths to carry out a role which neither on their own could achieve.

Shaun Webster MBE, who is a father and grandfather from Yorkshire, has a learning disability. Having previously had a warehouse job where he was bullied, he is now an International Project Worker at CHANGE. He travels all over the world to train professionals in inclusion, accessible information and independent living. As part of his work he works in partnership with children's rights charity Lumos, working as a mentor to young people in Eastern Europe who have lived in institutions. This was a kind of leadership which could only be carried out by a disabled person: "When they closed down institutions they were moving children back in the community. Children in institutions had no confidence and no belief in themselves. I was a role model. I trained them to have a voice, to be confident, to train other people with learning disabilities."

Shaun has diabetes (prevalent among people with learning disabilities) and contrasts the inaccessibility of information provided by the NHS, with support from a disabled colleague:

I wanted to do the right thing with my diet and so on but found I could not understand any of the information I was given. Catherine also from CHANGE was the one who helped me. She has diabetes as well as a learning disability and was able to support me by telling me how to spot the signs of problems with my blood sugars and explaining to me about diet in a way that I could understand.

A guidance or health coaching team with disabled members would be better placed to have an impact on the health of disabled people.

Every public service could identify roles such as inspector (peer), educator, befriender and advocate, that they would do better if the relevant teams included people who use services and family carers. Other functions, such as commissioning and planning could be done more effectively were some of existing budgets spent on resourcing local charities and community groups to input their expertise on what makes services feel more human. This would not only change those services, but would also tackle the 'them and us' attitude that has been fostered by our paternalistic or 'customer-focused' organisations.

Test Two: is every intervention future-focused?

One of the organising principles of our public services that I highlighted in Chapter Two is the distinction between preventative and reactive ('acute' or crisis) services. There is much talk and a few incentives for local areas to invest in prevention, but the legal duties on public services are to ensure that individuals who are in crisis receive the expensive, short-term interventions that remain seen as core business. Preventative or early intervention services tend to be funded with leftover money, which frequently runs out, and are run on a shoestring by voluntary sector organisations. The lack of money and planning involved means that these organisations are rarely challenged to demonstrate exactly what it is that they prevent or reduce, which is tricky in any case (how do you know what would have happened without the intervention?) and poorly thought-through interventions run the risk of hastening the dependence they seek to avoid.

An approach that focused on creating and maintaining wellbeing would remove the distinction between prevention and reaction: instead all services would promote people's resilience. Rather than layers of time-consuming assessments, there would be two possible kinds of offer for anyone approaching a support service: immediate crisis support for those who appeared to need it, or the help, advice and information needed to draft a 'wellbeing and resilience plan'. People in crisis would be offered that same planning support as soon as they could use it.

For everyone, the planning process would start with the same question, 'What does a good life look like for you?' before thinking about the ways in which the individual could achieve that good life. Where there was no obvious way of moving towards wellbeing and resilience without formal support, the planning process would consider the services necessary, but this would be after the individual and any family members caring for them had been supported to think about what they can or could do for themselves. In the next chapter I will outline the ways of doing this that already exist.

It is common sense that early and first interventions should focus where possible on resilience, but acute and crisis services can become future-focused, too, through intervening in a way that aims to build resilience, through leaving the individual better informed, more confident, able to access backup and better connected to those around them. Preventative services are widely regarded as having outcomes that are impossible to measure: what *didn't* happen. However, markers of an individual (or family's) resilience *are* measurable: we would measure whether people are well-informed about their condition, the choices open to them and the best coping strategies. People would report increased confidence, that they had access to emergency support and that they were better connected to others around them. These are all measurable proxies for wellbeing, which could attract payments where providers achieved them and penalties where they did not.

This unified expectation of building wellbeing today, with a future-focus on resilience and likely wellbeing tomorrow, would challenge even the most medicalised parts of the system. The psychiatrist who is brusque and cryptic, who ignores family members and prescribes medication without explanation may achieve clinical goals and symptom reduction if they are skilled at choosing effective medication, but they have missed the opportunity to build resilience and reduce the risks of a future crisis. Likewise, a surgeon needs not only to be able to carry out an operation skilfully, but to have the time and empathy to understand what the individual's goals in life are and what part an operation can and can't play in achieving them. That approach avoids the cost and suffering of unwanted operations, where for instance, an older person with a limited life expectation feels they will lose more from the disruption to their daily lives, than they could gain from medical outcomes.

Test Three: does every intervention connect people to each other?

Key to wellbeing and resilience is the extent to which people are connected with others. So, alongside achievement of their clinical or core goals, we should demand of all public services that they are delivered in a way that connects people to each other and avoids wherever possible disconnecting people.

Geoff Mulgan and colleagues have argued compellingly for a more 'relational' model of government and public service (Mulgan, 2010; Cooke and Muir, 2012). Connections between people were a goal of the personalisation reforms in social care explored earlier, but people who use personal budgets and cash Direct Payments can be even more isolated than those using traditional services, which at least put people together in one place. We should not lump people together in large buildings for the convenience of service delivery, but we can instead find new ways to connect people who need support, including those who take individual control of their budgets. Many councils have developed virtual e-marketplaces to enable their personal-budget holders to shop for support services, but few if any of those marketplaces enable those individuals to find others with similar needs, goals and interests, so that they can at the very least connect, but perhaps also form peer-support and advocacy groups, and in some cases pool some or all of their resources in order to exert more control or even co-design new kinds of support.

Connecting people should already be a mainstream goal of our public services, because we know that is linked to health, wellbeing and happiness, with isolation a serious health risk (Holt-Lunstad et al, 2010). If they were to be scored on their success in helping people to connect, we would see that a service that gives effective support or treatment, but which involves physically removing the individual from their home, may be less cost-effective than one with slightly weaker clinical results, but which allows the individual to stay at home and supports their relationships with their family or friends. The further and longer someone is taken away from their home, the less cost-effective the service is likely to be, compared to a viable home-based alternative. This is only a rule of thumb: where the family relationship has broken down, or someone can no longer safely care for a relative, then insisting the individual stays at home would do further damage, in which case, providing space and distance may be the better option. (But the value of even a troubled family relationship should never be assumed to be nil, permanently: where a positive family relationship can be re-established it is likely to achieve far more than any service and at far lower cost.)

Even services for people who live at home can disrupt their connections to others, through replicating or undermining support that was previously given by someone else, by forcing the individual to rearrange their lives around appointments (there are constant reports of home-care agencies who schedule support for older people to get up, eat or go to bed at antisocial or unpredictable times). Some services implicitly label an individual as 'different'.

Conversely there are many established ways in which services can help build and sustain social relationships or arrange their work around those relationships. Being located in ordinary buildings that are close to others in the community helps, particularly if those buildings are used by lots of different groups, rather than exclusively by one group. Small community enterprises bring people together into social groups. Where support teams include workers and volunteers who themselves have recent lived experience of a health condition, support relationships can be more reciprocal and lasting. Shared Lives and Homeshare are built as social models first and foremost.

A key problem for long-term support needs is that the people they work with require many years of support, but services, with their changing staff teams, cannot offer continuity over those timescales. On their own, they can be 'future-focused' only in the short term. Support networks, whether entirely informal or organised via a circle of support approach, can offer that continuity but currently have no status to interact with services, even if an individual wanted and asked for this. In British Columbia, circles models have been built on to become more formal 'micro-boards', which collectively take on legal powers on behalf of people with learning disabilities and others who lack the capacity to do so themselves. The new health and care system will need to find ways to recognise, build and work with the changing kinds of family, household and alliances that we choose to form.

Emotionally and financially sustainable families

The model of wellbeing I have described builds outwards from individual wellbeing, through supporting households, with the ultimate aim of creating change that reforms service systems and is felt within communities. Ensuring that people can live well as part of resilient households is a crucial step in creating this change. When we are in personal crisis, we find it harder to contribute to even those closest to us, which is an essential part of living well. Similarly, when a family or household is under unbearable pressure it turns inwards but, while many services talk of being 'person centred', most regard that person's family's wellbeing and success as beyond their remit.

Where services can be offered for the whole family, rather than treating each family member as an unconnected individual, they will be less disruptive of family life. In Māori culture, *whānau* describes a family group of parents, grandparents, children and uncles and aunts who lived together, were mutually supportive and had common ancestors. The concept of *whānau* has been developed in New Zealand into a kind of Family

Group Conferencing (FGC), a formal meeting where the extended family comes together to talk about concerns for a child who is considered at risk of harm or is breaking the law, and to find solutions together. The process now used in several countries is designed to include child, adults and professionals in a constructive way and to avoid confrontational and legal approaches to issues that do not require a more drastic child protection intervention. The concept of *whānau* has huge potential to be used by families or households who are caring for a disabled or older adult and the professionals involved in their lives.[1]

Thinking and acting whole-family would require a wide range of the health and care workforce to retrain and refocus. Ideally, they would need to be able to draw on specialists, such as family therapists, where the family dynamics are difficult. This will not necessarily be costlier, because it would reduce some of the time spent liaising with individuals separately, then unpicking the problems that occur when those individuals receive uncoordinated support. Some of this whole-household or group work could, however, be self-organising: many of us have become used to self-organising social networks with the aid of social media. A handful of social media applications, including Tyze and Rally Round, have been developed specifically to enable and coordinate support networks, while NextDoor aims to help neighbours organise activities such as neighbourhood watches. But using our emerging social networking abilities to develop more connected and social relationships between people and services remains largely unexplored.

Families are not only groups of people who share support needs, they are groups who contribute more in caring than the state. There are around 7 million family carers in the UK – around a tenth of the population – collectively caring for a large proportion of the people with long-term support needs on which public services spend so much of their time and money, with such mixed results. The government's offer to family carers is not in proportion to their £130 billion contribution (Buckner and Yeandle, 2015), consisting of assessments of need, the paltry Carer's Allowance of around £60 per week (2017/18 value), access to occasional breaks from caring for some, and information services. Local charities run patchily resourced Carers' Centres. But, because there are so many of them, politicians and service planners worry that increasing support to family carers would be 'opening the floodgates' or would lead to payments for what is currently unpaid care. (If we replaced Carer's Allowance with the minimum wage for family carers, the cost would be in the region of the entire cost of the NHS (Buckner and Yeandle, 2015). It would also bring employment laws and regulations into the heart of our most intimate relationships, with some fairly dark consequences.)

But if we stop seeing these families as just another group with support needs, and instead recognise that they take on, without prompting and often in hugely difficult circumstances, exactly the kind of self-supporting roles and responsibilities that politicians occasionally wish aloud that we would take on,[2] we would recognise that enabling families[3] to sustain their caring roles, while staying healthy and avoiding crisis, is self-evidently the most cost-effective use of taxes. With what would often be small amounts of flexible help, thousands of family carers would be able to stay in at least part-time paid employment and avoid spending years on out-of-work benefits.

The debate between government and campaigners often boils down to how much carers should be entitled to in benefits and breaks. But perhaps more impactful would be to share the resources, knowledge and respect currently reserved for those in paid service roles. A rule of thumb would be to look at everything people in paid caring roles can access – training, induction, equipment, a team around them, emergency backup – and consider whether it should and could be offered to unpaid family carers. Some of this would have little cost, such as enabling family carers to take places on existing staff training courses, or providing easier routes to specialist knowledge and experts. At present families carry out technical and medical caring tasks without the proper information and training in how to understand and use those medicines, equipment or interventions. This can be stressful, ineffective or even dangerous.

At present, carers talk about trying to fit in as many questions as possible when they meet consultants for scarce and brief appointments. Instead, health services could take a collaborative 'wiki' approach to ensuring that reliable information is generated and available where it is useful, alongside the availability of experts with enough specialist knowledge to field questions, whether face to face or via phone and online. Providing support of this kind would require services to refocus and could need more investment in specialist information provision, but would reduce the resources needed for crisis responses.

Equipment, whether it is expensive and technical, such as lifting equipment, or simple and cheap, such as grab rails, can typically only be sourced by family carers via a tortuous and time-consuming process of assessments, referrals and procurement. These administration costs are incurred because services do not trust families to make sensible requests. That lack of trust is insulting to people who have often taken on far more responsibility, unpaid, than the well-paid professionals doing the rationing. Where families can plan for a good life and can see how to achieve it, they do not typically ask for the earth. There are countless examples of families winning control of their health or care budgets and then proceeding to design support packages which cost a fraction of the unwieldy and intrusive state services they battled to replace.

In a system that did not render families invisible, taking on an unpaid caring role would give people access to a commensurate budget for aids and adaptations, from companies (licensed where the nature of the equipment required it) with whom they could deal direct. A small charge per item would do a great deal to reduce unnecessary orders, in comparison to an entirely free system. Where someone's requests were large or unusual, that could trigger a further assessment conversation or visit, but these interventions would be reserved where there appeared to be a significant unnecessary expense, not where someone was in danger of getting one more grab rail than might be essential. This is another area of state support where the safeguards against fraud or poor decisions cost more, directly and indirectly, than the waste they are designed to guard against. Few people want to make their homes look like hospital wards unless they really must.

Carers UK regularly estimates the amount that carers contribute to the NHS. But there has been surprisingly little effort to calculate the obvious costs to services, tax revenues and the welfare state of caring roles becoming unmanageable alongside paid employment, or becoming unmanageable entirely. An even more hidden cost is that of the growing number of people who simply opt out of caring unpaid for often distant family members, prioritising their careers, childcare responsibilities or both. If both the value and the hidden costs to the whole system (NHS and social care, benefits bill, tax revenues) of our current model of family caring were clearer, we would probably conclude that one of the first goals of our support services should be to enable families to remain emotionally and financially sustainable. This is not the same as the present approach of fending off families for as long as possible while their caring roles increase, until they reach breaking point. The most cost-effective approach for the whole economy would be to invest in family carers to incentivise more of us to take on part-time caring responsibilities, while protecting us from all-consuming caring roles where possible. This clearer contract between state and family in which responsibility was shared, recognised and rewarded would give people confidence that taking on a caring role was not inevitably a one-way street to unemployment or ill health.

In the current system, the level of support a family receives is hard won (through months of demeaning assessments) but easily lost forever. The quickest way to be denied or lose support is to offer to do the caring yourself. So as mentioned in Chapter One, any improvement in the individual's independence, or any increase in the willingness of the carer to care, is not met with any positive reward from the state, but with a reduction in support or personal budget. For people with fluctuating conditions such as multiple sclerosis or mental ill health, this is particularly difficult, but it is frightening for any individual or family who makes a potentially fragile recovery: if the situation deteriorates again, the previous support will take months to regain, during which the family will remain in desperate circumstances.

The solution to this is to give families the ability to retain for a short period their entitlement to any service (or personal budget) that is reduced when things get better. This could be done in two ways: one would be that the family's entitlement to resources would remain in place for a fixed period after those resources have been reduced or withdrawn. If the family's need increased again, they could re-claim the original level of support without going back through the assessment process (which would also reduce administration costs). Alternatively, a portion of the savings made by withdrawing the resources could be put into a notional contingency fund, held by the council or NHS, which the family could then draw on in the event of an emergency. Either system would incentivise families to experiment with less state support, without feeling they were risking an unmanageable crisis.

This principle could be extended still further. At present, families are told there are no resources to support them with their home-based caring. But if caring unsupported proves unmanageable, then a hospital or institutional service might be put in place, which can cost thousands of pounds a week (in the case of adults with learning disabilities and mental health problems for instance). Only service managers can access those very large amounts of money, not families. A simple solution to this would be to oblige service managers to tell the individual (or, with their permission, their family or advocate) how much money they are intending to spend on an institutional service and to give the family an opportunity to put a cheaper solution in place themselves. This is already possible, using existing Personal Health Budget regulations. Some families would only be able to do this by consulting with a community-based service and asking that service to manage the budget, rather than managing it themselves (again this exists: the Individual Service Fund). Rather than obliging the family to prove their proposal was 'safe', the onus would be on services to demonstrate that their more expensive, institutional solution was better for the individual.

I have outlined some possible changes to make support services think and act whole-family, but those changes would also need to be matched by changes in employment rights that recognised caring for adults as being as important to us and to society as caring for children. It is not feasible or sensible to force caring roles on anyone: to do so would violate the rights of the person being cared for, not just the carer; but in time, our own attitudes to family caring would change if we found ourselves able to make a wider range of choices about how much caring it felt sustainable for us to take on.

From customer service to shared responsibility

The changes outlined in this book would bring new rights to individuals and families to shape their own care and services. But they also imply a clearer sense of our responsibilities. For unpaid family carers, the responsibility is already there, just not fully recognised. But for others, including many who live within the health and care system for many years, responsibilities are not just the price of having rights, they are integral to those rights, because without responsibilities we are not full citizens.

This attitude change won't be easy. Whether we work in healthcare or not, we are all taught that health professionals know best. The expertise of our health professionals, based on years of training and incredible advances in research and medical technology stops suffering and frequently saves our lives. But that attitude of 'doctor knows best' is less useful when we feel that we aren't really responsible for our own health, or can't manage our own care. And it can be lethal when the health system ignores the insight of people themselves or their families.

Earlier I outlined the problems with being a public service 'customer': we will often have few of the choices available to customers and little or none of the buying power. But even if those things were fixed by a better-funded and organised public service system, the more fundamental problem is that the relationship we are looking for from the people who support us is not, at heart, a customer relationship. For many of the quarter of the population living with a long-term condition, some of their key relationships will be with the people who work for their support services. Choosing who those people are is a good start to establishing a positive relationship with them. Being able to choose a service that is 'high quality', staffed by well-paid and highly trained workers, can also help. But Shared Lives carers are not particularly well-paid and many do not have qualifications, and yet they appear to be able to help people live well and achieve more, because they have a relationship with the people they have chosen to support that is nothing like a customer service relationship. It is more akin to the relationship that family carers have with their relative, and carers are another group of people who often achieve astonishing things without any of the resources or trappings of the 'high-quality service'.

Through joining or remaining part of a family or household, the people in Shared Lives, like many people cared for within their own families, are not just recipients of care. They contribute and they share in the responsibilities of the household. We cannot live confidently as citizens if the spectre of illness or simply old age looms over us, threatening to bring financial or physical ruin because services are either prohibitively expensive or simply not there when we need them. But equally we cannot live as full citizens if we are forced to give up our responsibilities towards ourselves and others as soon as we develop ongoing support needs.

At present, there is a lot of excitement in the health service about 'self-care' and 'patient activation'. Patient activation is the field of trying to help and encourage people with long-term health conditions to take more responsibility for managing their health. There is a patient activation measurement (PAM) system that tracks the extent to which people are taking responsibility for their own health, managing medication and 'self-caring', rather than relying on medical professionals. 'Activated patients' are likely to be living more healthily and experiencing fewer health crises.

Patient activation is a great example of how trying to add the right thing into the wrong system creates at best uneven and imperfect change, and at worst can mutate into another problem. If you start by thinking about people with long-term support needs as patients, who need to be activated by doctors, you've already lost. Patient activation is reminiscent of the terms, 'compliance' and 'non-compliance', which refer to whether you take the medication your doctor wants you to take.

So what would be more helpful formulation of this agenda? Looked at through the person's eyes and those of people closest to them, not through a professional or service lens, an individual with a long-term condition is not primarily a patient: they are living their lives – sometimes their whole lives – alongside a health condition, but their aim in managing their condition is not to be a good patient, but to live well. The key NHS contribution to that good life will be the provision of information, support, medication and kit that promotes health and wellbeing, but this will only translate into living well when the system as a whole (health, care, housing and not-for-profit organisations) is designed around informing, empowering and connecting people.

So as presently formulated, the PAM is likely to impact that which it seeks to measure, and may do so negatively, through framing the wrong kind of relationships. What we really need to measure is the extent to which people and professionals have an activated relationship: a clear, shared idea of what wellbeing looks like and clear individual and joint roles in pursuing it. The individual will be acting outside of the implied job description of 'patient' and the professional will be thinking and acting beyond their clinical goals. So we need to measure not just how activated the 'patient' feels by health professionals, but how activated health professionals are in pursuit of wellbeing.

The new system designers

Some poor or partial implementations of 'transformed' or 'personalised' public services have simply replaced one set of problems with another. Whereas before unaccountable public service bureaucracies failed to treat people as individuals, some systems have now created systems in which predominantly large, private sector organisations enjoy monopolies. Those organisations were supposed to be more 'customer focused', but in reality, repackaged familiar services with new branding while cutting costs. This happened because decision-making power was moved from one set of managers to another, never towards the people who use services and their families.

Talk to people involved in planning and delivering public services and you will meet people whose job titles and responsibilities for budgets suggest that they have power, but rarely will you find people who feel they have it. Service users think the professionals they come into contact with have power over their lives. Front-line workers feel they are working within the restrictions imposed by senior managers. But those senior managers feel powerless to close the gap between their vision for better services and the stuck reality and cannot understand why front-line workers and middle managers remain stubbornly unreachable and untouched by their vision. We can locate the problem in our politicians but as any junior government minister will tell you, the first lesson of government is the apparent impossibility of change.

So there is no shadowy 'them' who have power over 'us'. Our public service systems are only 'us': the sum of the beliefs and relationships of all of us involved in them or touched by them. So 'we' will make change happen, or no one will. That means that 'we' will have to comprise a different mix of people.

This shift from 'them' being responsible for designing as well as delivering public services, towards us sharing that responsibility, has become known by the clunky term, 'co-production',[4] intended to distinguish collaborative decision making from consultation. Consultation often means saying, 'Here's our decision; what do you think?' or, more insidiously, 'Here are some options we've chosen; what do you think?' (when in fact the cheapest option has probably already been decided on). Co-production is the combination of two collaborative activities: the first is co-design, in which people are involved from the earliest, 'blank sheet of paper' stage of planning and throughout. The second is co-delivery, in which people who want to be, continue to be involved in delivering the service or intervention. This involvement can mean mutual or peer support, it can mean a role in reviewing what is working and needs to change, or it can (rarely at present) mean creating employed roles that are made open to people who use or have used the service and value their lived experience alongside other skills.

People who use services and their families are often 'represented' in local public service decision-making committees by the director of a local charity and someone who has personal experience of using the service. But these representatives are there on sufferance. The expert by experience is usually untrained, unpaid and has no mandate from others, while everyone else around the table is a paid professional, secure in their status and remit. For real co-production, decision-making bodies must resource user-led organisations, who then elect representatives. Planning teams will include salaried employees who have current or recent lived experience.

This idea will appal some in highly paid management and commissioning jobs. Their work is so technical, so demanding, so *difficult*, that it couldn't possibly be delivered by the kinds of people their services support. There is some truth in this: their jobs as currently conceived would be undoable for most of us. But they are also undoable for them, no matter how talented they are. A very senior and successful public service manager, faced with cuts, spiralling demand and constant regulatory imperatives, told me, "I have accepted that my job is undoable, which is the only thing which keeps me sane. All I can do is use my position to protect my team from as much of the crap as possible."

There will always be a need to manage complex budgets and balance books, but if that is the *only* skillset well-represented in the planning and management workforce, then service decisions will be based around the best short-term use of currently available financial resources, ignoring whether outcomes are being achieved and making little or no use of assets such as the people who use the service, volunteers, family carers and community groups. At present, in the UK, groups of senior finance professionals tend to be mainly white, male and middle-class, which further restricts the breadth of their views.

There is a small number of national co-production groups of people with lived experience and family carers. One of the longest standing is the National Co-production Advisory Group (NCAG), which is a key constituent of a national partnership aiming to support social care services to become more personalised, called Think Local, Act Personal. Through NCAG people with lived experience sit on a board alongside representatives of central and local government, the NHS, professional bodies and representatives of care-provider organisations. The partnership has produced guides, training and other kinds of help for councils and provider organisations that want to make their social care provision more personal and human. This collaborative approach to policy making belies the usual view of government policy making as being a battle between ministers and civil servants on one side, and lobbying groups and charities on the other. Despite the many problems in social care and the lack of money, co-production resulted in the

Care Act 2014 which enjoyed a remarkable degree of consensus and which is written in unusually plain English.

In a meeting which included a minister and NHS England's CEO, I saw the impact that people with learning disabilities, employed in meaningful roles by CHANGE, could have on a moribund conversation. As mentioned earlier, the Winterbourne View scandal at an Assessment and Treatment Unit (ATU) for people with learning disabilities and medical (usually mental health) needs, uncovered scores of similar institutions flourishing in a hinterland between social care for people with learning disabilities and medical care for people with mental health problems. ATUs are ostensibly for short-term assessment and 'treatment', but up to 3,000 people with both learning disabilities and mental health problems were languishing in ATUs, some of them for years, at a time when most thought that institutional care was history. 'Experts' like me had accumulated thousands of meeting hours and report pages, talking about familiar kinds of improvement: quality, safety, training. The 'improvement programme' had been a top priority, with the minister's personal backing. The work was urgent, so reports, quality schemes and guidance were produced at breakneck speed. The urgency meant that there was no time to involve people with learning disabilities in producing those resources, which takes time. That fast pace, however, was illusory. Three years on, there had been no progress whatsoever in reducing the numbers of people living in medical institutions.

The ministerial 'summit', organised by people with learning disabilities from CHANGE and other user-led organisations, had a very different tone from the previous three years of meetings. The people with learning disabilities who spoke at the meeting were polite, but much blunter than their non-disabled counterparts. For most people involved in the post-Winterbourne View change programme, the abuses at Winterbourne were horrifying, but not personal. Most were non-disabled and did not have a relative with a learning disability. In meetings, particularly stressful national meetings in front of ministers, we (people in leadership roles), who generally know each other well, look after each other. We have invested a lot in our long-standing professional relationships.

For the people from CHANGE, however, the people experiencing poor care were like them and their friends, who had almost all experienced inexcusable care at some point. They were not thinking about their future professional relationships. They had a unique moral authority to demand change. They did not understand jargon, so people were forced to at least attempt plain English, which probably meant that we all understood each other more clearly than we usually do. They chose to focus the meeting on the need to employ more people with learning disabilities in the learning disability sector: its support services, training programmes, advocacy services and inspections. I had not heard this idea raised once in the years of previous meetings on how to 'improve' things, but their reasoning was that nothing fundamental would change until non-disabled workers were forced to see people with learning disabilities as colleagues, not just as patients or service users. They also rejected the idea of 'improving' medical institutions: they demanded their closure.

One meeting did not change the world, but it did for the first time leave ripples in the previously unperturbable face of a system that had been causing misery and harm too often to too many people. Without the right people moving at the right pace, everyone had rushed off in several wrong directions.

The organisation I work for has since recruited people who use Shared Lives to our team as (part-time) paid colleagues. They talk in public about Shared Lives, health-check local services and drew up a charter for what good Shared Lives should look and feel like. They do these things more effectively than we could before. But just as importantly, my colleagues and I have needed to stop thinking of people with learning disabilities always as the people we help, because some of them are now colleagues.

The role of personal budgets in redesigning the system

As one professional described the impact of introducing self-directed support approaches in substance misuse treatment:

> It's created an equalisation of power, as they are doing their own self-assessment. They're telling you things that they wouldn't have told you before.

> You're spending more time with them. There is a
> lot more care that goes into this care plan. It has
> opened our minds, so rather than just banging them
> into rehab we're looking at the full picture. (Welch
> et al, 2013: 24)

Some on the left have argued that personal budgets are incompatible with a collectivised public service system and welfare state: an opt-out from a failing system that would not be needed if the system was better. In fact, used well, personal budgets can be the greenhouse in which the new system is seeded and starts to grow. This does not happen frequently at present: personal-budget holders are largely ignored by service planners who continue to focus on the bits of the system they continue to fund or purchase themselves. One reason why personal budgets are not always embraced by service planners and managers is because they cannot see how budget holders can be anything other than a drain on their scarce resources, 'fracturing' traditional services or making them even less economically viable.

Of course, where people make genuine choices, sometimes they will not choose to use existing services. This makes some services, particularly those that are tied to a big building, unviable. A half-empty day centre or care home will go bust and close, to the detriment of the people who still want to use it. It is hard to argue, however, that people should continue to have to use (and sometimes live in) services that are not what they would choose. Services are supposed to sustain people who use them, not the other way around. Money in the system is finite: there must be some closure of services if new ones are to start and grow.

But personal-budget holders could be brought back into the system, connected with each other and with those who retain budget management powers for local councils and the NHS, so that data about what they buy, and would like to buy but can't find at present, can be fed back into the service design and review process. Personal-budget systems do not remove the need for commissioning, but they do change how it happens, with input from personal-budget holders becoming a key part of the commissioning process. Commissioning teams in turn, would need to employ people with experience of using services and others who could understand and make the best use of that insight.

From protests to public service movements

The NHS in England appointed three organisations in 2016, the New Economics Foundation, Nesta and Royal Society of Arts, to lead a programme called Health as a Social Movement. Its first report (Del Castillo et al, 2016) notes how extraordinary it is for a major public sector leader, NHS England Chief Executive Simon Stevens, actively to call for social movements within his domain, given that social movements are by their nature grass-roots, messy and keen to challenge those in power. Stevens recognises that the challenges of achieving health, as opposed to fixing illness, require there to be social movements towards healthier behaviour that will both reduce the numbers of people needing NHS care and reduce the demands on the NHS of those who are living with long-term health conditions.

This idea of shared goals between people at the very centre of power, and those who are at the coal face, is a departure from the more familiar campaign or protest group, which springs up in opposition to a public service or government failure, but that typically remains firmly outside the system it criticises, rather than seeking to share responsibility for redesigning and co-delivering a different system.

NHS England under Stevens has been supportive of several grass-roots campaigns led by front-line staff, such as the We Nurses group. The various change and 'grass-roots' campaigns receive communications support and backing from enthusiastic senior leaders, but the limitations of social movements and bottom-up change in effecting change to core public service activity are taken for granted by everyone involved. The limited expectation of progress is evident in the way the system interacts with and supports these campaigns: there is great interest in how they start, and in how they can be encouraged and enabled to change the behaviour of 'patients' and of front-line workers, but no sense that front-line behaviour change will progress up the line into less comfortable territory, such as how the people within these movements might take control of budgets or whole services. So, I have witnessed many genuinely warm relationships between very senior managers and activists who may be junior workers or 'service user activists', despite these activists calling for radical change. Both activists and senior leaders share the view that 'the system' gets in the way of the change they would both like to see. Both may scratch their heads at the way a heap of middle management layers and budgetary controls lie, untouched, between them. With the key levers of money, targets, inspections and performance management all continuing to pull in the direction they always have, it is 'the system' that continues to mandate unchanged behaviour from middle managers, rather than the activists' appeal to humanity or the senior leader's 'vision'.

The children of Sharon and Patrick Terry were diagnosed with pseudoxanthoma elasticum (PXE) in 1994. With no relevant experience, they self-trained and sought the help of researchers to identify and patent the gene responsible for PXE. Sharon went on to found several organisations and alliances dedicated to furthering genetic research into rare conditions, including The Genetic Alliance, which encourages families to share genetic information, by putting them in control of their participation in research. Linked initiatives also enable families to share information with each other, to crowdsource reliable evidence and to form their own campaigns and support networks, which have now spread internationally.

Sharon is truly exceptional, but for more grass-roots movements to lead to real and lasting change would require the mechanisms to be in place for a genuine transfer of money, resources and power from their current loci, towards movements that successfully articulated a different world view. All public service organisations can redesign their decision making to seek, collate and analyse the messages gathered from staff, service user and family carer networks, and build the representation of those networks into their governance structures. If service leaders shared some of their internal and external communications resources, these decentralised learning networks would become a key source of leaders at every level, which could be integrated into staff development and training programmes. People who were active in a network, whether front-line staff or people who used the service, would be given access to training and development opportunities, on the assumption that some would be the best candidates for employed roles within the organisation, including taking on positions of power themselves (which would carry the inevitable risk that they became the next generation of bureaucrats, of course).

The need for a slow policy movement

The only kind of change you can make happen suddenly, on a large scale, is destruction, whereas creation of anything real and valuable starts small, but ambitious. For real change to take hold, you need to involve people who don't always agree with each other and you need a tolerance for messiness: the neater the plan, the more fictional it is. So public service leaders need to be willing to draw on the expertise of people who use their services, and from grass-roots movements, but ultimately, we may need to replace our existing power structures with decision making that feels more like those movements: collaborative, decentralised and human.

At present, government and the NHS express the importance of a policy change through the urgency of the deadlines they set themselves and their partners and the amount of money they can 'find' in an emergency to fund the change. As in the post-Winterbourne View example, or more recently in the NHS Sustainability and Transformation Plans (STPs) which every area has been ordered to produce, important decision-making processes are frequently handed to small groups of very senior people (or sometimes suitably expensive consultancy firms). These groups will exclude large parts of the relevant sector, particularly its smaller and messier charities and grass-roots groups, which are complex and time-consuming to find and talk to. People with lived experience and their families, who would need training, preparation and a slower pace in order to contribute meaningfully, will be consulted in brief sessions if at all. The senior people or consultants on their six-figure salaries will say, without irony, that their budget is too tight to fund deeper 'engagement' work. It is no surprise that STPs, despite many containing necessary and pragmatic ideas, have been widely reported by the media as 'secret NHS cuts plans'.

Where new approaches are piloted, there will be rushed evaluations whose findings can only be tentative, due to the small numbers and short time periods involved, that recommend that further research is needed. By this time, the crisis will have become the new normal and the sense of urgency will have dissipated. Committee reports and research evaluations will lie unused. Pilots will quietly close, as the public service sector resumes business as normal until the next crisis.

This cycle of crisis, frenzied activity and shallow changes is endlessly repeated. The urgency turns out to be illusory every time: while a report will be rushed out in months, underlying causes of problems will remain unaddressed for years. The abuse at Winterbourne was merely the latest in a succession of abuse scandals stretching back to the 1960s, and continuing today. STPs are morphing into the next set of initials while the NHS and social care continue to go bust. The next 'never again' scandal will be along soon.

The model of change I have presented in this chapter is not a 'culture change', which no one sees as their responsibility and which probably will never happen. But it does take time: months rather than days to recruit, train and employ people with recent lived experience to co-lead and deliver change programmes, inputting their own expertise and meeting with others who don't want such deep involvement, but who have insight to offer.

There is a slow food movement, which began in Italy, based on the belief that fast food lacks real nourishment and flavour and that its intensive production methods and shortcuts are unsustainable for the environment within which it is grown and produced. Slow food is produced with time, care and the understanding of local culture, farming and ecology, which can only be developed over years, or even generations. It tends to value small-scale production for its sustainability and for being rooted in community and place. Carl Honoré (Honoré, 2005) argued for this philosophy to be applied to many areas of life and Peter Bate (Bate, 2005) applied it to the practice of inclusive decision-making.

We need a slow policy movement in our public services: a new norm for how to create change. No more flurries of reports and plans from the same group of highly paid people, who will remain embedded in the group-think that brought them to the crisis in the first place. Instead, the slow policy approach would be to cultivate different people and networks which are more deeply rooted in the lives and service cultures of those affected: people with lived experience, their families and front-line workers. A change programme would examine the problem or challenge from the point of view of people use services, families, front-line workers and people who do not or cannot currently access the service. The conversations with them will start with 'What does a good life look like?' not 'How can we improve, cut or close replace our service?' The questions will include, 'What are you willing to contribute to achieving the goal we all agree is important?' (which is a different question from 'Will you pay for our service?' or 'Will you volunteer for us?') In place of short-term pilots generating tentative findings, new models should be implemented on a small scale but with a plan to scale them up incrementally if they appear to be working, until they replace the current system. With the people who use services genuinely involved in their design and delivery, we would finally have the confidence to remove resources from models that do not work, rather than continuing to resource the status quo, regardless of how much more effective new models proved.

The alternative is to do what we have always done and get what we always have.

Escaping the invisible asylum: actions

1. Make the goal wellbeing
The goal for any public service should be achieving wellbeing now and developing the resilience to hold on to it.

2. See assets as well as needs
Look only for needs and they are all you will find. Our services need to be able to see, value and build on people's assets and those of their family

and community. The group designing services will need to be as diverse as its local communities, to be able to recognise everything that those communities want, and can offer. Confident services are clear about the resources that they bring and how they can work alongside the capabilities of the person and their family and friends. Recognising what people can bring is not just limited to how people can organise their own personal care, but how they can help to co-design whole service systems.

3. Think about the future as well as the present
In the moment in which most people approach services, their needs and problems are easier to spot than their capacity and potential. Meeting 'presenting need' is only a partial success: real value for money comes from intervening in a way which is likely to see the person happier, more confident and more independent in the future.

4. Connect people
If our close relationships are key to our wellbeing and resilience, it follows that public services should connect people to others and avoid at all costs disconnecting them. Achieving wellbeing for people and value for money for services usually means ensuring the individual remains part of an emotionally and financially sustainable family or household.

5. Move slowly to move fast
Whether it's getting to know an individual in order to help them plan a better life, or getting to know a whole community in order to design more accessible and welcome services, investing time in understanding people and what they can bring is never wasted, whereas time spent introducing ungrounded change programmes often is. A truly decentralised and collaborative model of public service management will first enable everyone to act with individual autonomy, but will then help people to connect with each other to share responsibility for the resources available to them.

EIGHT

Delivering the national health and wellbeing service

Too often, we offer people a service, when what they are looking for is a relationship.
(Richard Jones CBE, former adult services director)

Valuing what we've got

Implicit in the proposal to create a new kind of health and care service is decommissioning at least parts of the current one. It is worth restating that this book should not be read as a charter for cutting state services. Services have already been cut beyond the level at which real suffering is being caused to hundreds of thousands of UK citizens, including the 1.2 million older people who need state support but are denied it (Age UK, 2017). We need all the current investment in public services, and more, if we are to catch back up with the hugely increased demand for support, much less keep pace or overtake it. So we still need most of our current institutions: our hospitals and care homes and prisons, but if the changes in this book reduced demand on them, they might return to something like sustainability. In other words, building a new system is a matter of survival for our traditional services, not a case for their closure.

One of the ways in which we need to change our view of public services is our tendency to think of a building, such as a hospital, as a public service and therefore treat the whole collection of resources in and around that building as one, inviolable public good. A hospital, school, nursing home or community centre is a collection of kinds of resource, which include the buildings, the kit in those buildings, the services based in them, the staff teams and the capacity of the people whom they support. All have value, but their relative values are not all equally recognised within public service hierarchies, which value resources according to the proportion of the overall budget they account for. So the most powerful people in the system manage the largest budgets.

Also contained within and around any building are the relationships between the people who use it and work in it. Those relationships do more to determine the effectiveness of most services and their impact on people's lives, but they are invisible and have no cash value. There is no senior manager responsible for them. They might be thought of as transitory, but in fact they can outlast the kit and sometimes even the buildings themselves. They are a kind of a community, and it is in its community that any support service holds its memory and accumulated knowledge, not in its files and records.

The people in these buildings – both those who use the services and those who work in them – are also part of a local community. The resources of those communities are ultimately crucial to the success of what happens inside those buildings and services but they too sit outside of the service's budget lines. We need to be able to see and value all of those kinds of resource and the interconnections and dependencies between them. Only then will we be able to combine community and state resources in new ways.

Community and how to build it

So building communities is not an alternative to sustaining public services, but investment in communities and public services needs to be seen as inextricably linked, with investment in communities taken much more seriously than it is at present.

Politicians and other leaders sometimes talk as if 'community' is a semi-mythical beast we dream of tracking down and snaring. But community development work is not that mysterious: it has been established and researched for decades by the Asset-Based

Community Development Institute and other bodies, with dozens of manuals.

In the process outlined by John Kretzmann and John McKnight (1993), successful community building is asset-based, internally focused and relationship driven. It starts with mapping a community's assets: finding the people who want to contribute. Some just wish to take part in occasional events or conversations; others through taking the conversation to others or even being employed as community builders themselves. This approach was used by the Royal Society of Arts Connected Communities programme which found that even communities that were commonly thought of deprived, depressed and lacking in social capital, contained people who were thought of by those in their neighbourhood as the person to approach for advice or help. Its reports (Rowson et al, 2010; Marcus et al, 2011; Parsfield et al, 2015) argued for programmes aimed at strengthening community action to look for existing community resources and relationships and build on networks of relationships which were valuable but often incomplete.

For instance, during the miners' strike in the 1980s, women had become heavily involved in organising support for the strikers, such as meals on the picket line and food and other assistance for families who were slipping into poverty during the extended strike. Some of these women had been using their talent for organising and problem-solving for years and were seen decades later as the go-to person by people who found formal services intimidating or confusing. In some communities, these 'community catalysts' can sometimes be postal workers, shop owners, hairdressers or people with milk rounds or other roles that brought them into regular contact with otherwise disconnected people. Some people in these roles build up trust and naturally start to help and connect others, developing a word of mouth reputation for helpfulness. Typically, they are invisible to the state or seen as a nuisance, rather than a resource. Few have strong and constructive relationships with the system, limiting their ability to create change. An organisation called Unlimited Potential in Salford takes an asset-based approach called 'positive deviance', in which community workers, faced with an apparent problem, look not for the people experiencing the problem, but those who do not, in order to identify what causes some people in the same place and circumstances to stay well, connected and resilient, enabling those people to be the catalyst for change in others. One of Unlimited Potential's groups is Salford Dadz, which tackled a widespread local issue of fathers in the community becoming disconnected from their children and families, sometimes following family break up. They found that dads who did not fit that mould tended to be more emotionally open, so they involved them in social groups with dads who were having problems, which in turn led to a huge range of social and health benefits for a group who had previously been thought of as 'hard to reach' and 'disengaged'.

By 'internally focused', McKnight and Kretzmann meant that the solutions to the community's problems lay in its strengths, not in outside agencies, which have the tendency in the dominant deficit-focused model of 'helping' communities, to take up the resources allocated to those communities, paying for their staff, offices and resources, whereas for McKnight and Kretzmann, that money would have been more effective going directly to people and the community itself.

'Relationship driven' refers to the idea that, because the key assets of a community are the people and associations within them, the key challenge of a community building is to 'constantly build and rebuild the relationships between and among local residents, local associations and local institutions' (Kretzmann and McKnight, 1993: 9). The Connected Communities programme found that 'Social relationships have a value ... through working with communities this value can be grown by connecting people to one another in their local areas' and argued that 'investing in interventions which build and strengthen networks of social relationships will generate four kinds of social value or "dividend" shared by people in the community'. These are a wellbeing dividend, a citizenship dividend, a capacity dividend and an economic dividend (Parsfield et al, 2015: 7-8).

The asset-based community development (ABCD) philosophy reverses the usual view of problems as being within communities (particularly the most 'deprived') and the solutions being outside. This model has led to much successful community development work, but that work does not always have a clear view of how it will include people who have significant physical-, social- or health-related barriers to participating in their communities, nor of how they can become not just as participants but also potential leaders. And while the literature provides a powerful challenge to paternalistic services it has less to say on what those services should do differently, beyond getting out of the way.

The learning from Shared Lives and other approaches is that it *is* possible to combine productively the strength of communities, the capacity of individuals who need long-term support and the resources of a nationally scaled and regulated service. Asset-based values can and must be embedded within public services, and this starts by recognising the humanity of both people who use services and the people who work for and manage them.

Forming human connections has relied in the past on face-to-face contact and the telephone. Much has been achieved by circles of support, self-advocacy and user-led organisations, and grass-roots networks, like Partners in Policymaking, that have built networks of people who use services and their families, and also started to build bridges between the worlds of formal and informal care. But the internet and social media offer a new way for our chosen networks of friends and supporters to overlap and connect with each other and, if we choose, with a new kind of public service.

New interventions

The new health and care interventions we need can be roughly divided into new ways for people to approach and access support, and new ways of offering that support itself.

A new front door

Public services are torn between whether to keep people out, or to drag them in and keep them there. Social care has tied up too much of its precious resources in a gatekeeping system that requires ever more proof of dependence and poverty to let people in. It's like an exclusive nightclub with huge bouncers and an unfathomable door policy, but once inside it is disappointing and hard to find your way out of. The NHS's front-of-house primary care services, with their easy access, highly trained and often heroically conscientious GP gatekeepers, are unable to cope with the flood of people desperate for help that is either woefully scarce (your friendly GP can make a referral quickly, but the specialist is months away) or outside of the remit of any health service (the lonely older people who have nowhere else to go for human contact). Mental health services can offer easy access to a self-help manual or short course of brief talking therapies, but require you almost to have the noose around your neck before more specialist care will open its doors. And once through those doors, it can be difficult ever fully to find your way out again, or they can become the 'revolving doors' orbited by the growing proportion of people who experience more than one diagnosable condition at once. At the end of the line await our care homes, with their one-way entrances.

The new way in to public services needs to reject the notion of fortification, and to do so just as the number of people gathered on our services' borders and crammed within their refugee camps seems unmanageable. We need many more ways in to public services, which are easy to find whoever you are and easy to enter, because when people really need the asylum of intensive support, they need it rapidly. They will not be guarded, but they will be staffed by people who have the time and freedom to help people make choices. Those choices will include but not be limited to state services as the first or only option. These entrances must also be exits: leaving a service's domain may be just as urgent as entering it.

Some areas have become enthusiastic about the idea of single front doors and one-stop-shops. This is admirable, in its attempt to create simplicity, but also has drawbacks. It is difficult for a single information and assessment service to be equally accessible to everyone and to be staffed by people who understand the full range of needs and wishes that people may come with. It can look messy and expensive to commission a multiplicity of information offers for a single area, with dozens of small grants or contracts given to local charities, each with their area of expertise or community of interest. But rather than rationalise them into one information service, it would be simpler to adopt a single purpose and success measure for all information providers. Like the rest of the system, their single purpose should be to enable people to achieve and maintain wellbeing.

To facilitate this unified approach, we would need to be able to take ownership of our own medical and other service records. The wellbeing and resilience plan would be a single transferable support plan, which we owned and shared with professionals we met, as we chose. This does not have to be a national IT project (there is a long history of failed projects of that kind): it could simply be a shared format, given to each individual in paper form if they wished, or via email, for them to share with whichever services they chose. Third-party IT suppliers could offer a vault service in which individuals could store records, with the individual encouraged to give access to services with which they were in contact. Individual services could retain backup records of the information they had collected and a copy of the plan they had contributed to.

Patients Know Best, founded by Dr Mohammad Al-Ubaydli, offers a 'patient controlled record' to people making extended use of the health service: their health and care information, which they can share with whomever they trust and which connects with wearable activity devices and tracks signs and symptoms. It works on any computer with no software needed and enables people to choose to share their data with researchers if they wish. Through ceding control to the individual, clinicians, services and researchers ultimately gain access to more information, but on the citizen's terms, not theirs. It is used by thousands of people.

The idea of starting a person's interaction with public services with an easy-access conversation with someone whose job is to inform, empower and connect people, with services as the last, not first, resort, is already being put into practice in 13 UK areas using Australia's extensively evaluated Local Area Coordination (LAC) model. Local Area Coordinators (LACs) combine a range of traditionally separate roles (advice, community development, community social work) and are embedded in local communities, working alongside children and adults who are disabled, have mental health issues or are older, and with their families and communities. LACs are funded by and employed by the state, but sit on the borders of community and services, as these accounts from Thurrock's LAC programme evaluation illustrate: 'The individual was receptive to the LAC where he hadn't been in the past. This was due to the LAC's persistence and also the fact that he wasn't a health professional' (Sitch, 2014).

There are several keys to an LAC's success: they can intervene early and are free to talk and listen, rather than 'assess needs'. They focus on 'staying strong' and connected (and can keep that focus when working with people who already use services but want to become less dependent and more connected with their community). Whereas an early decision for many professionals is, 'Is this person eligible or ineligible?' an LAC does not have to make that choice and can therefore work across service and eligibility boundaries:

> Before the LAC had been introduced to Mr R all he did was sit indoors 24 hours a day. The LAC has provided opportunities for Mr R to get out of the house a lot more involving helping others. Mr R's Psychologist ... commented that she had seen a drastic improvement in Mr R since working alongside the LAC and she felt he had stayed well for longer than she had seen before, avoiding a crisis and potential admission. (Sitch, 2014: 13)

> I now know who to go to if I have a problem – it used to be so difficult to find the right person or I'd have to wait until my problems were even worse before someone would listen. (Broad, 2015)

Another individual who required crisis response and out of hours services 41 times over a seven-month period, consequently made three calls over the next four-month period in which they were working with an LAC. The 'demand reduction' can be achieved because those involved do not approach their work as 'demand reduction'.

This approach opens no floodgates: LACs help people to build their own resilience, not their use of services, and even to add their own social capital. LAC has the potential in the UK to replace a chunk of our expensive and ineffective systems of social care assessment and gatekeeping. Working with and within GP practices, LACs could provide support to the legions of lonely older people and people with long-term mental health problems who take up a large proportion of many GPs' time, despite there being no possible medical solution to their problems. For instance, a woman of 88 was referred to her LAC by her GP, who had noticed that her GP appointments were increasing and felt this was not for medical reasons, but due to isolation which had worsened following a bus service closure. The LAC helped her to build more links and activities in the community, and to approach a community organisation which ran a community bus service. Her increased support networks were felt to be key to her quick return home from hospital after a heart attack and the LAC helped link the community organisation to colleagues who supported it with a successful bid for a new community bus service.[1]

The change in approach, can help to drive a deeper change in the aims and focus of public services: 'The change in thinking since working to the Local Area Coordination principles cannot be underestimated. For all involved there has been a mind shift and constant challenge to how we "do business" and how we work with people and communities' (Sitch, 2014: 6).

Similarly, social prescribing is a way for GPs to link people who come to them with non-medical problems, or problems that do not have a wholly medical solution, with interventions which are also non-medical. GPs 'prescribe' a wide range of social, exercise, food or lifestyle activities delivered by local organisations to people who could benefit from them. In the most developed models, those organisations which are well used and effective receive a share of NHS funding or infrastructure support. Social prescribing is a way to use the universally accessed nature of the GP practice to reach people who may approach no other service, but rather than insisting on a medical response, or drawing the person towards formal state services, the prescription can a way to direct people back out to the community, with support which is more likely to be of benefit to them.

Jen Hyatt describes the common purpose of the 30 health-related social enterprises she has been involved in founding over many years as giving people the tools to enable them to live the life they choose. This applies to her new ventures, Troo

Life Coach and Eartime, as well as to Big White Wall (BWW) which she exited in 2015. BWW was set up to offer people who were 'anxious, down or not coping' with a safe, professionally facilitated online space where they could access information, take courses, self-assess, gain or offer peer support and speak live to a therapist. BWW was accessible 24/7, anonymous and free via the NHS in many areas. It did not replace mental health services (although Jen says we need to 'decommission loads of crap which does not work'), but it offered people the choice of a low-risk way to explore informal and formal support at their own pace. It was offered to millions of people via the NHS, Armed Forces, colleges/universities and employers.[2]

Jimmy Wale, the founder of Wikipedia, drew heavily on the work of Friedrich Hayek, an economist who famously asserted that knowledge is dispersed among the members of society, but unevenly so (Hayek, 1945). So, a central committee is unlikely to be the best decision-making body, but relying on the 'wisdom of crowds' might lead to large numbers of uninformed views outweighing the informed ones. Wikipedia has created more than 40 million articles in more than 250 different languages, used by half a billion people each month. Its collaborative approach to editing has resulted in a large proportion of its articles being highly accurate and well-referenced, allowing readers to check the veracity of the information they read. It is not flawless: articles on recent events or grounded in recent research, as well as articles on controversial subjects, often contain errors. Knowledge within public services is also highly unevenly distributed, with great reliance on experts, which makes information provision expensive and patchy, as well as vulnerable to the gaps in knowledge or mistakes of those experts. This is one of the many challenges facing GPs, who are expected to be experts on a dizzying range of health (and sometimes non-medical) concerns and treatments, in a world where research is producing new insights and debunking old ones at an accelerating rate. NHS Choices is a large web resource of verified medical information, which is a useful resource for those aware of it and able to access it, but its information is necessarily static and conservative, whereas much of the knowledge from which people could benefit most would be personalised and interactive.

Partners in Policymaking, a loose, powerful network of hundreds of disabled people, families and workers, uses the simple, almost archaic approach of people phoning people they know, who phone people they know, to track down information that can be otherwise unavailable to them. A number of the disabled children and young adults in families whose parents were part of the network were facing serious medical problems related to sitting in a wheelchair. They had the 'windswept' appearance of being hunched over to one side, which most people would assume was part of their disability, but was actually a side effect of sitting in the same position all day, every day. The combination of muscle weakness and posture was resulting in organs being put under pressure and in some cases people were undergoing multiple major operations to address what had developed over years into life-threatening medical problems. The parents could not access specialists until their children's problems were already acute, but through sourcing and sharing information they were able to establish that there were simple preventative interventions – such as placing a rolled-up towel in the right places when someone was lying down – which could be used to correct postural problems before they resulted in a crisis. This was knowledge that they had gleaned from their contact with specialists, from online forums or through their own research. There is clearly a risk to information of this kind, but there was also a very significant risk in not being able to access information. In this instance, the economics of having an easier route to a specialist, or of recruiting more specialists in response to the unmet demand, would make sense for the health service which would avoid thousands of pounds of complex and often dangerous operations.

Could a networked approach be used to create new routes to specialists, or to collate information about unmet need so that resources were directed where they were most needed? There are currently over 500 groups of stroke survivors meeting with support from the Stroke Association and other organisations. Diabetes UK has nearly 400 groups for people with diabetes. Macmillan supports 900 independent cancer groups. There are tens of thousands of others for major and rare conditions. These groups currently may have no access to specialist expertise, despite offering the opportunity for highly cost-effective communication. A purely decentralised 'wiki' approach to information would contain too many risks of misleading information causing serious harm, but if we could use networking approaches to combine information produced wiki-style, advice from trained experts by experience and the deployment of fully qualified experts, we could significantly increase both the value and accessibility of information currently held too unevenly.

The principle behind these approaches is not to ignore people, or their needs. It is not to 'signpost' them endlessly to dwindling and overburdened services that direct them on to the next service which can't help, or park them on a waiting list. It is just enough information and advice, offered by people who have got to know the individual well enough to have a good idea of what 'just enough' looks like.

For those who move on from the information and planning stage to take up a formal service, rather than making 'customer service' offers, it would be more realistic if taking up a service's support for anything but a brief period of time was framed as an informal contract, with expectations and responsibilities set out clearly on both sides. The purpose of doing this is to create clarity about what can and cannot be achieved, and to build trust and cooperation. Some of these 'contracts' will be broken by the people using support, but it will be vital to resist the temptation to build in the penalties and sanctions of a legally binding contract: more would be lost in doing this, through the creation of fear and mistrust, than could be gained. Most people, when they are clear about what a service can do, its limitations and what the people involved need from them, will make some attempt to play their part, and if they could do so, the gains and savings would be huge.

Through the front door

If we apply the previous chapters' design approaches (co-design with people who use services, front-line workers and families) and tests (Is it asset-based? Is it future-focused? Does it connect people?) to the support-delivery element of a new, wellbeing-focused health and care system, it is clear that interventions that are currently small and peripheral will need to become the core of the new system.

In British Columbia, a version of Shared Lives is used by more than half the people with learning disabilities who receive accommodation and support, in contrast to the UK where the three areas using the model most have reached only 10% of people with learning disabilities who need support. No model should be imposed on people (which some critics would say has been the case in British Columbia), but if Shared Lives only reached 10% of people with learning disabilities nationally, this would amount to 5,000 more people, saving around £70 million a year. Cheshire West offers Shared Lives to the greatest proportion of older people at 2.5%; every area catching up would see another 14,000 older people receive short breaks, day support and extended support (Shared Lives Plus, 2017). With more ambitious goals to offer the model routinely to people with mental health problems, older people and other groups currently rarely offered Shared Lives, tens of thousands would move from care homes and other models into Shared Lives with immediate savings of hundreds of millions of pounds a year, with huge additional gains from improved health and wellbeing.

Other models, such as Homeshare, the community or microenterprise home-care approach and Buurtzorg (discussed later in this section), have proven their value sufficiently on a small scale to make a strong case for national investment. Together they could also be used by hundreds of thousands of people. Given the financial, quality and safety problems now besetting the current health and care system, the onus should not be on successful new models to prove that they deserve a greater share of the available resources, but on existing models to prove why they do not.

Many of our existing services will still be needed however, and some providers of them have already shown that they can pass the three tests and realign themselves around the goal of individual and family wellbeing.

I have referred to a few of the stream of reports finding problems and failures in the home-care industry and outlined why the economics of home care make it increasingly difficult to aim for anything higher than the bare minimum of support, with even that low bar not always being reached. There are home-care providers that buck that trend. For instance, Home Instead services consistently achieve 'good' and 'outstanding' ratings. CQC inspectors praise its ethos of getting to know people as individuals, tailoring care and its strong links in the local community, such as one service manager's delivery of dementia awareness training to the public – including bank and shop staff – to help them understand how to help people with dementia that they come into contact with. Home Instead is a global franchise, with the resources to develop consistent training, for instance, but local responsibility for delivery. Providing consistently good home care is possible, but most of the agencies doing so are marketed at the wealthier among people who have to buy their own care, rather than being available to state-funded care recipients.

One successful change within home-based care is the development of 'reablement': support to an older person (usually), designed to enable them to get their independence back following a stay in hospital. Most older people in England can access six weeks of reablement for free, but only a few initiatives have extended its ethos into longer-term home care. Wiltshire council developed an initiative in which people could continue with their home-care provider after the six week period, or switch to another, depending on the provider's performance, which combined individual choice and the council's close monitoring and challenge of its providers, in an attempt to improve performance.

Age UK has developed a 'Personalised Integrated Care' model, in which older people who are living with long-term conditions and are at risk of recurring hospital admissions can access coordinated voluntary, health and care support. This is one of the few initiatives that attempts to address medical, practical and social support needs in a coordinated way. Evaluations suggest it works and it is being adopted by an increasing number of areas.

In the radically devolved Dutch Buurtzorg model of home care, an experienced nurse coordinates a small team of colleagues, organised and self-managed on a peer-to-peer basis. The team provides a highly personalised combination of care, navigation and coordination. The model costs more per hour but has demonstrated that it results in people requiring half the hours of support, through helping individuals and families to build their resilience, support networks and caring skills. The highly autonomous nature of the small, self-organising teams of practitioners rests on in-depth recruitment and selection processes, combined with an ability to be self-policing within a small group in which people know each other well and share a sense of ownership and responsibility. Buurtzorg claims that people require around 50% of the usual hours of care and the overall cost is 40% cheaper, saving the Dutch government around €2 billion per year.[3] The approach flies in the face of accepted wisdom about how services 'scale up', but has grown in under ten years to support 70,000 older people (RCN, 2015). A Scottish home-care organisation is attempting to remodel its entire offer on Buurtzorg and it has inspired Wellbeing Teams, developed by care expert Helen Sanderson, which several areas are currently developing.

Similarly, some care homes have rejected the 'end of the line' model, where a closed dormitory sits behind a neatly manicured lawn, to become community hubs, housing a range of services and developing shared use of gardens and communal spaces (Mason, 2012). Some of the best care homes, according to CQC, pursue a different ethos. They actively seek the views and opinions of people living in them, and their families, as guides towards doing things better, rather than seeing those views as 'demands' on their time. Peregrine House, an 'outstanding' home in Whitby, explicitly seeks to replicate the care that would be provided within a family, and involves family members in activities such as Zumba, which are adapted so that those who cannot stand can still join in. Another outstanding home was described by residents' relatives as 'treating you just like family'. Just as oppression and neglect can become normalised as staff are desensitised to their effects, in Peregrine House, the positivity and warmth become self-reinforcing: rather than organising the team's work around the basic tasks of feeding and the toilet, owner Kevin O'Sullivan says, "In a lot of care homes, that's their raison d'être. It takes all day. We say to the staff – we all have bodily functions, they don't take up your day. Let's get those things out of the way and then spend time with the residents doing nice stuff" (Smith, 2016).

In Cornwall, Perran Bay Care Home is also outstanding. CQC said,

> What makes Perran Bay care home special is its extremely strong links to the local community. It is at the centre of the village, it is the largest local employer and the whole community interacts with it. In return Perran Bay offers work experience, apprenticeships, hosts community events, and supports local businesses. (Healthcare Leader, 2015)

The people who manage and work in these care homes are taking a social as well as a caring approach to social care, despite the lack of financial incentives or regulatory or commissioning insistence on doing so. How many more people who have chosen to work with people in the caring professions would follow their lead, given slightly different circumstances?

GP practices can also become community hubs: a collaboration of primary health, mental health and voluntary sector services which are designed to respond to the mixture of medical, mental and social issues which people bring to them. Altogether Better works with practices interested in developing a new model of care to deal with the rising levels of demand from people whose health and wellbeing needs cannot be met by a clinical intervention alone. They support these practices to find enthusiastic people who are willing to give their time to work alongside the practice as volunteer practice health champions. The champions are not given a predesigned role based on what the practice wants, they are supported to develop their own ideas based on what motivates them. Citizens work together with the practice: no longer seen just as 'users or choosers' of services but as 'makers' and 'shapers' of new services that are a better fit with people's lives. In turn, people use their services differently.

Robin Lane Practice in Leeds now works with over 50 people who organise groups and activities ranging from a ukulele group to seven-days-a-week breastfeeding support. They also constantly update a directory of local services and resources. This has tackled intangible issues like loneliness but has also resulted in hard financial and clinical outcomes: the Saturday flu clinic is attended by over 800 people, up from 300. The practice has increased their patient list by over half without any increase in referrals to either primary or secondary healthcare services and a 10% reduction in use of the Emergency Department. Robin Lane has been willing to be shaped by local people even where this leads to changes that some would see as inappropriate to a health service: it has a bar and an open mic night, weighing the risk of promoting alcohol use against the bigger gains of becoming a place in which the community spends time and of which it feels real ownership. By late 2017, Altogether Better was working in over 120 GP practices.

Most national leaders will conclude from the small scale of these initiatives that they are nice but not significant. Could they become the norm? They feature better staff pay, training and ratios, which are not funded by most state procurement. But they also increase wellbeing and health, draw in unpaid contributions from the community, and some have lower management costs and staff turnover. Without the economic, regulatory and ownership reforms discussed later, they are likely to remain outliers which show us a tantalising glimpse of what the people who work in and use care and health services, with help from their families and communities, could and would achieve if they were allowed to.

Working in the new system

The eminent thinker and disability rights activist John O'Brien describes the rise of a mechanistic view of service provision in Wisconsin, which he sees happening globally. Pressure on service finances and the desire to rationalise and merge care provision results in the 'cogworld story' of how long-term care should work:

> People need long-term care because they are
> incapable of performing activities of daily living.
> Long term-care efficiently and cost-effectively
> performs the specific tasks that people have proved
> that they cannot. These tasks are specified in a
> plan that links objectively assessed incompetence
> to procedures that are well defined for efficient
> performance. Whenever possible long-term care is
> delivered in a person's family home, especially when
> family members and friends can provide unpaid
> assistance. As need becomes more intense people
> move into specialized settings: assisted living, group
> homes, nursing homes. (O'Brien, 2015: 11)

It is hard to see an affordable solution to the problems O'Brien
and many others identify, using employees in care-work roles as
currently defined. It would simply be too expensive to enable
professionals to spend enough time with the same individual in
order to build up positive relationships. If we spent hundreds
of millions of pounds to double rushed, 15-minute home-care
visits to 30 minutes, the older person would still spend the vast
majority of their day alone.

When people describe receiving really great ongoing support,
they will usually talk about the relationship they have with that
individual, and it will be one that does not stick rigidly to a
job description, but in which the worker has gone 'above and
beyond' their duties and feels more like an ally or a friend than
a contractor. If great support work feels like having a friend,
why not create support roles that are designed to create real
relationships, rather than hoping that people will take personal,
financial and professional risks in order to behave more like
humans than their current roles suggest is wise?

Employed models

The directly employed personal assistant model outlined in
Chapter Five cuts out layers of bureaucracy and involves a
very personal relationship between a disabled person and the
people they choose to employ. The balance of power, which

would otherwise be transmitted from a large organisation through the pressures it placed on its staff, shifts to the disabled person, often with very positive results. A new risk arises, of the disabled person exploiting their new power and their workers (particularly where workers are migrants or rely on their employer for their accommodation) but UK reports of this are not widespread. Friendships between an employer and their employee carry risks that disabled people have had to learn to navigate, but the reciprocal nature and shared interests of these personal relationships have their own protective power in most circumstances. Similarly, the very small-scale nature of the care and support microenterprise model that Community Catalysts has developed, replaces investment in inflexible bureaucracy to create consistency and manage risk, with the added value and flexibility of personal relationships. People working in microenterprises are often self-employed, which tips the balance of power more towards them (in the absence of any exploitative middleman), but the quality of the relationships can be similarly positive.

Self-employed models

The recent 'gig-economy' cases show the risks of self-employment within industries that do not value people: large commercial service-industry organisations want the control and rigidity of an employment contract, with all of the flexibility and the low-cost base of self-employment, depriving workers of pay and their basic rights. Genuine self-employment relationships are characterised by meeting a number of tests, which include the self-employed person being able to choose who to work with, where and when they work, and having freedom to make decisions within their role. So, self-employment works in Shared Lives because the Shared Lives carer chooses with whom to share their life; they work flexibly (doing activities that they and the individual both enjoy and going on holiday together, for instance) and they work from home and in the community.

Shared Lives carers, like Buurtzorg workers, are carefully recruited and can access training, breaks and support. The national models for Shared Lives contracts aim for fairness and autonomy, within the broad structure set down by the role description and each individual's care plan. Their commitment has boundaries and a contract, but they are free to form lifelong attachments in which both parties regard each other as a friend and genuinely 'just part of the family'. As outlined in Chapter Six, this does not lead to greater risks of abuse, but to consistent, long-standing relationship and far fewer safety concerns: CQC consistently rate Shared Lives as the safest form of adult social care.

Shared Lives shows that self-employment within structures which balance consistency with flexibility can work for both parties. To make the less boundaried time commitment of Shared Lives attractive and non-exploitative, matching supporters with individuals (and their families) becomes an essential part of the support planning process: Shared Lives carers give so much time because they spend a lot of it doing things they enjoy with people they enjoy being with. The Shared Lives approach is akin to social franchising, in which a central agency creates the framework of rules and boundaries into which individuals or small groups can fit their own personal expectations. Social franchising would be one approach to scaling up the microenterprise models without losing the creative individuality of the enterprises.

Effective and ethical self-employment models require more investment in recruiting and inducting support workers, but reduce the costs of performance managing, sanctioning and replacing failing workers. Some of the savings in the Buurtzorg model arise because there are no leaders within the teams and, after induction using a coaching system, individuals work on the basis of consent and a web-based patient information database which is used to organise the different roles in the team, build the formal and informal caregiver network and share information and best practice. The lower costs of management enable higher front-line wages and job satisfaction is indicated through its unusually low sickness rates. Astonishingly, the national team has fewer than 50 employees to support 6,500 nurses in 580 autonomous teams; the overhead costs are 8%, compared to the average of 25% despite the challenging nature of the work: half the 70,000 people supported have some form of dementia (RCN, 2015).

Buurtzorg has inspired SuperCarers, one of the increasing number of internet-based start-ups, which invests time and technology into rigorous recruitment of skilled support workers, then uses internet technology to enable people to choose and rate compatible workers. These models also tend to include GPS monitoring in order establish when a worker was present at an individual's house in order to automate billing, and Trip Advisor-style ratings so that people can see how others felt about each worker. By keeping the costs low, these businesses are able to pay self-employed workers a higher wage, which could make it easier to attract better staff.

Most of the internet start-ups attempting to be the 'Uber for social care' use a self-employment model, but people working for start-up CareShare, which matches people and caregivers, can choose whether they want to be self-employed or pay into employee benefit schemes for the security of employment. CareShare is also a co-op, owned by both workers and people receiving care and people who receive care can choose to offer support or services to others and be rewarded through a time-banking approach.

There are varying levels of organisational involvement and mediation in those relationships, from the entirely unmediated relationship between a disabled person and the PAs they recruit themselves, through more mediated models in which brokerage agencies vet, recruit and help to monitor, to models like Shared Lives, in which self-employed people are recruited rigorously over a period of months and then matched carefully and continue to be monitored while nevertheless working with a great deal of autonomy.

Self-employment lacks the job security of an employment contract, but if people are genuinely self-employed – able to communicate directly with people who can directly engage their support – this could bring much more continuity for those workers who are highly valued than short-term or zero-hours contracts. They will also no longer be at the mercy of the funding relationships and finances of a central organisation. Just as people who use services are most empowered when they have individual rights *and* the opportunity to form alliances and partnerships, so self-employed workers would have the opportunity to associate into informal support networks, form limited liability partnerships, or become part of structured entities like Buurtzorg.

Peer support and family care

The most plentiful, but also least well-supported, source of long-term support is unpaid: the UK's 7 million family carers. I have already outlined how the role of unpaid family carer could be much better valued and supported, not to attempt to load more responsibility onto those million plus people who already take on heavy caring roles, but to enable more of us to take on sustainable part-time caring roles, while maintaining our health, sanity and any paid employment. With such large numbers involved, collectively contributing scores of millions of hours of support, small gains in the sustainability and effectiveness of those roles would make more difference to our health and care economy than almost any other change.

Alongside the contribution of families, many people who have support needs themselves already contribute to their own care and to that of others. It is getting easier for people who share a health condition or disability to find each other and form peer-support networks, some of which are supported by charities while others are self-organised entirely on the internet.

One of the most wasteful aspects of the current system is that the people it supports include many who would like to – but cannot – get into employment and volunteering. Peer support is rapidly being established as an effective approach to helping people to build their own wellbeing as to be part of a mutually supportive group. While behaviour-change programmes have often focused on information provision, research suggests that people quickly reach the limit to which they can take in more information and reject much of it in favour of beliefs which are rooted in their experience and emotions, and therefore insusceptible to being changed purely by information and rational argument. They are much more likely to be influenced in their behaviour by their peers (Burd and Hallsworth, 2016).

Peer-support programmes are usually small and assume that peers will only be involved on a voluntary, unpaid basis. This suits many, who may not have the health or time to take on paid roles, but there has been little serious exploration of the extent to which people with lived experience could take on existing paid roles that could benefit from their insight and empathy, such as some of the thousands of information-giving, care-planning, advocacy and health-education roles. This would create new role models for people using services, affecting their view of their status within an organisation and fostering a shared sense of responsibility, as well as enabling people with long-term conditions, who experience high levels of unemployment, to move into paid work, building their skills, experience and confidence. For some groups using services, this shift is achievable now, within current resources. For more systematically excluded and oppressed groups such as people with learning disabilities, it would require investment and ambition on a generational timescale, starting with the education of disabled children. However, organisations like CHANGE have shown the potential for disabled people and people with their own long-term support needs to take on paid roles as well, as peer-educators, trainers, inspectors and befrienders.

Volunteers and time banks

Up to 3 million people regularly volunteer in some form related to health and care services, and almost half the population volunteer in some way at least once a month (Naylor et al, 2013). This social action is already worth £34 billion to public services. £10 billion of this does not show up in formally recognised volunteering, but takes the form of people helping others (beyond their relatives) and community activity. Yet service managers regard volunteers as a source of unskilled labour, delivering 'nice to have' rather than essential roles and social action is 'not yet central to the way most services are planned, commissioned and delivered' (Clarence and Gabriel, 2014: 13).

Wellbeing-based public services would clearly need to invest in social action, to offer a more humanised response and to tackle areas of wellbeing such as participation in community and tackling loneliness, which they could not otherwise address. Social action would remain a parallel approach to more formal services, but could also be embedded into how many services themselves are delivered, with much more coordination of paid and unpaid roles. Effective investment and planning could unlock many billions in additional value, given its multibillion-pound contribution.

One risk of services attempting to embrace social action is that they stifle it. At present, voluntary agencies typically recruit, train and deploy their volunteers in similar ways to their employed workforces and imbue them with the same hierarchical culture and the division between people who support and people who are supported. Charities still talk about their 'beneficiaries'.

However, social action development can move away from the 'gift model' and aim for reciprocity and equality. North London Cares and South London Cares hold social events and match up young professionals with older people who might otherwise be isolated. The two organisations recognise that they are tackling loneliness that affects both generations, not just the older people. The Homeshare model brings together older and younger people who can help each other in complementary ways.

Time banking, which can be traced back to nineteenth century socialists and was rediscovered by Edgar Cahn in the US in the 1990s, (Cahn and Rowe, 1992) enables people to value and exchange unpaid contributions of time, so that people can both give and receive help, without being exclusively in the position of giver or beneficiary. Someone offering support is offered an equivalent amount of another time-bank member's time in return. Spice has built a time-credits model, which draws in local businesses who donate hours (an hour at the bowling alley, swimming pool or football club for instance) and links with local charities who need hours of help. Hours can be taken in the form of paper one-hour notes ('time credits'), which can then be saved, spent in other areas with similar schemes, or gifted to others. This is not just a neat way to get more people to help each other: it benefits the people who take part and changes their relationships with local services. Spice's surveys of the 30,000 people who have earned time credits found that nearly two thirds felt better informed about services, but that did not mean they were necessarily using more formal support: a similar proportion said they felt both healthier and more socially connected through participating. A third said they visited the doctor less. Nearly half were giving their time in social action for the first time.

Most of us feel distinctly uneasy about unpaid volunteers providing intimate care, or vulnerable people relying on unpaid volunteers who have no legal obligation to work. Volunteering or other forms of social action cannot and should not replace services, nor should services attempt to subsume people's desire to help each other into their existing, medicalised goals and world view. Shared Lives services demonstrate that it is possible to combine the safeguarding or value-adding aspects of a public service with social action, but there are tensions in doing so. These come out for instance, when risks are taken which may feel ordinary in the context of family life but over which service systems feel they should have control. Services will only be able to benefit fully from the vast potential of social action when they are willing to reshape themselves at least partly in its image, sharing their resources and their power to define what 'good' looks like.

Measuring what does and doesn't work

Earlier I argued that most research funding is provided to research the most widely used services (which can also provide large populations to sample), not the small and innovative ones, generating an endless feedback loop of increased evidence about traditional services and forming a barrier to replacing them with innovations. So commissioners gain a false sense of security purchasing a 'proven' intervention, while less-used interventions remain seen as risky, despite many small-scale evaluations.

Rationalising the goals of public services into one set of wellbeing goals presents the possibility of measuring a single set of outcomes in comparable ways across a wide variety of kinds of established and new public services. At present, the clinical outcomes expected for an individual in a hospital ward are well established, but no such measuring of outcomes apply to people using most community and social care services. Those tools and surveys that do exist do not generate data sets that can be cross-referenced against each other. With one set of outcome measures, whether an individual was currently in a hospital ward, a care home, a Shared Lives household or in their own home, their achievement of wellbeing could be measured and contrasted with similar people using different models. Something like this happens in education: every school is measured against the same attainment measures. The Justice Data Lab makes reoffending data available to organisations rehabilitating offenders, so that even small charities can tell whether they are meeting or exceeding expected rates of reoffending for the individuals they support.

The new public services can start with small changes designed by people and front-line workers, but only if the same outcomes are measured across the existing and the emerging system. These cannot be time-limited pilots followed by evaluation reports. It is astonishing how many pilots are funded with no plan to move resources from current 'core' work into their continuance and expansion if they work: failure is built into innovation. Instead, innovations should be tested and evaluated as they go along, with the commitment to increase them gradually if they appear to be working, thus generating more evidence and more opportunity for refinement. There is something to draw from the research and development (R&D) approach of innovative private-sector organisations: rather than waiting for absolute proof that never comes, as it becomes clearer that something appears to work, investment is moved from what was the norm, to the new approach. Rather than the current ad hoc allocation of funds to pilots, it would be preferable to mandate that every public service system have an identified R&D budget.

Academia itself would benefit from a similar shift in power and decision making to the one I have set out for public services. Research is planned between senior managers and senior academics, with little reference to the views of people who use services and front-line staff. The bigger and more established the service, the more power its managers have to negotiate with academics and the more influence they wield with government research budget managers. Some public-service-facing universities have 'user' and 'stakeholder' reference groups.

A smaller number are developing peer-researcher models in which people who use services are trained and supported to carry out research, moving away from the fantasy of the dispassionate, neutral academic and instead recognising that every researcher is human, and that a mixture of backgrounds and insights are the best guarantee of a grounded view of an intervention's impact. But every university that researches public services with public money could actively involve people who use services, families or front-line workers in identifying, prioritising and designing their research programmes.

A couple of small think tanks are trying to do this. CoVi (Common Vision) aims to make its research and learning widely accessible, through using visual communications such as animations rather than traditional reports. Guerrilla Policy aims to crowdsource ideas for where its work should focus and to develop a network of engaged participants who help to resource, carry out and disseminate its messages.

This book does not just suggest a new set of services, but a whole-system transformation. It is difficult to research or model the many interdependent and complex impacts of whole-system change. As we have learned from the personalisation reforms in social care, partial implementations of whole-system changes will always bring deeply contestable results so, arguably, the only way to test it is to do it. Even then, the interdependent nature of a set of linked changes makes them almost impossible to subject to any study with a control group, or to attribute cause and effect.

All we can be sure of is that the current system is *not* the right one. We know – and it is not disputed – that despite everything that medical science, technology and other advances have achieved, our system excludes unacceptable numbers of people, generates unacceptably high levels of failure, and is going rapidly bust. Set against those certain failures, we know that we need to take risks.

Measuring what doesn't work

One way to manage and mitigate the risks of any public service system, would be to measure both the positive and negative impacts of services. Tools that measure both the positive and negative outcomes of support exist but are rarely commissioned by support organisations, which are keen to demonstrate only their positive impacts to their funders. While medicines are tested for side effects, public service interventions are assumed to have only positive impacts.

Services would typically see measuring their negative impacts as an attack on their effectiveness, but they would be wrong to do so. It is only by understanding and weighing up the positive and negative impacts across a broad range of a person's wellbeing indicators that a service can be confident in what it is achieving and clear about what it cannot. At present, our public services present a take-it-or-leave-it offer. A clearer picture of the trade-offs would allow a more informed choice on both sides of whether a service was likely to help deliver the life that a person wanted, the role that the service could play, and what the risks were.

This would also present an entirely new opportunity for public services to improve. At present, improvement is only possible through achieving greater positive outcomes, or cutting costs for the same outcomes, not reducing the likelihood or impact of a service's unmeasured side effects.

This would also transform risk assessment and management culture, providing a framework within which managers and practitioners could more realistically support risk-taking by the people they support. So for instance, in taking a hospital discharge decision, instead of a one-sided picture, in which the risks of the person's home were listed exhaustively, but the risks of being in hospital entirely ignored, the risks and opportunities of both would be weighed up, making it more likely that a practitioner would feel able to countenance a support package at home, whereas at present any risks of that are compared to the pretence of perfect safety within the hospital ward.

Paying for the new system

Despite the savings identified through the lower cost and more effective models outlined earlier, it bears repeating that, following years of unsustainable budget cuts, no new health and care system can cost less than our current one. The gains would be in health, wellbeing and happiness, not tax cuts. In a wellbeing-based system, money will still be a key concern, but not the only concern, as money becomes one resource to be considered alongside others, including the expertise and contributions of people with support needs themselves, the unpaid contributions of family carers and the resources of the wider community. With all of those resources valued in terms of their role in creating and maintaining wellbeing, it will be possible to establish some equivalence between very different kinds of resource and intervention. A small community group may never be worth as much as a hospital, but it is worth something. The key challenge is not to develop ways to value intangible assets, but ways to pay for the wellbeing- and resilience-related outcomes outlined earlier.

Existing clinical measures remain important, but where two interventions can achieve similar clinical outcomes, additional wellbeing measures would show that an intervention that informs, connects and empowers people, or one that adds 'social value' is more cost-effective than one that relies entirely on paid staff or takes place in an isolating building.

Alongside paying for these positive outcomes, it would be important to penalise reductions in wellbeing and resilience, to disincentivise 'failure demand' (the demand for further services which is a result of a service's failure to achieve outcomes) and incidences of repeated need.

The closest things we have to payment systems that reward wellbeing are the Accountable Care Organisation (ACO) models, imported from some healthcare insurers in the US – notably Kaiser Permanente – who make more money if they help insured people to stay well rather than having to provide expensive treatments, and so have developed end-to-end support systems, with early interventions and outcome-based care. Where preventative interventions can be shown to work, they are invested in and care is provided in the least expensive appropriate place, reducing reliance on hospital buildings and keeping more people at home.

An ACO is a lead service provider organisation (or a more equal 'alliance' of several) that takes on responsibility for the health and wellbeing of a whole population. The contracts pay organisations for the support activities they carry out, but there are additional rewards and penalties for achieving or failing to achieve a set of outcomes. The outcomes require all of the health, social care and other organisations to work together, so organisations are incentivised to cooperate and think holistically about people's use of the whole system, not just one service. So far, ACOs remain promising but rare, struggling with the politics of organisations working together for the first time and the legal and regulatory complexity of forming new working arrangements. Some ACOs have included charities and community organisations in their new partnerships, with promising results.

Australia's new National Disability Insurance System (NDIS) aims to personalise support for working-age disabled adults and takes a similarly system-wide view of cost-effectiveness. Its designers have attempted to combine individual tailoring of support with the macroeconomics of managing budgets nationally. In the UK, attempts to devolve budget control to the individual level are constantly undermined by financially driven attempts to micromanage and often cut those personal budgets in order to reduce local care budgets. Each individual is treated as a separate budget line to be cut, resulting in expensive, bureaucratic and adversarial care planning processes and precluding longer-term or whole-community investment to build the wellbeing and resilience that would create lasting savings. The Australian system is run by an agency that is challenged with balancing its overall budget, potentially giving it the flexibility to approve preventative and resilience-building interventions, providing that they are genuinely effective in helping people to achieve more independence and therefore result in lower spending overall.

Moving to a truly outcome-based payments approach across our health and care system would be complex and fraught with risks, as it transferred risk around a system already at breaking point. It would be possible to create a shadow system of measures and notional payments to model the potential impact and to give organisations the opportunity to realign their activities, before moving to a live system.

Owning the new system: the future is mutual

Taking the arguments on empowerment, co-design and co-production to their logical conclusion, were public services to be genuinely shaped around the capacity and responsibilities of front-line workers and the people who use them and their families, most service providers would be co-owned by those people.

Co-operatives UK have highlighted the small number of organisations that are bringing mutual ownership into care and support (Co-operative College and Change AGEnts, 2017). I mentioned CareShare earlier. Choices4Doncaster has brought some of Doncaster's small care providers together into a cooperative, while Cartrefi Cymru, a co-op providing support to disabled people in rural Wales, has over 200 members drawn from workers, care recipients and the community. Its chief executive, Adrian Roper, lists the benefits of its reciprocal relationships and greater community participation but also that the current 'arms-length' procurement approach, in which 'people's support is commodified' into 'a static number of "need-hours"' which are sold to competing contractors (Sheffield, 2017) is an active barrier to their approach, with councils likely to regard new cooperatives as riskier than less-imaginative models.

An idea running throughout this book is that a key determinant – perhaps the most important determinant – of the success of a long-term support arrangement is whether it creates and maintains the conditions in which real and reciprocal relationships can be formed and sustained between everyone involved. None of the mainstream ownership or governance models are fully compatible with this. Statutory services tend towards bureaucracy. Private-sector services embed a customer relationship culture that promises more choice and control than it can deliver and that inherently does not want to share either its resources or its power. Charities often have 'gift model' thinking at the heart of helping their 'beneficiaries'.

Adopting mutual ownership as the default governance model for public services could be an important part of embedding the kinds of shared-responsibility relationships that lead to more cost-effective support. There is an opportunity to build on existing but tentative government legislation that has created theoretical rights for staff teams or community groups to challenge councils for ownership of certain public services. The *Localism Act 2011* established the principle that community organisations should be able to challenge councils for control of public services, through putting in a bid to take over and run a service. However, moving to genuinely mutual models could not be achieved purely through imposing new legal forms. NHS Foundation Trusts are technically already a kind of cooperative, with staff as their members. Some governors must be 'the public', but patient membership is discretionary. In reality, this model amounts to occasional consultation. Public service 'spin outs' have enabled services that were previously tiny parts of large bureaucracies to become stand-alone social enterprises, with varying degrees of shared ownership, but those new organisations have to compete, often against the private sector, in a lowest-price market that does not put a monetary value on their values.

One way of achieving genuine mutuality, evidenced through co-design, opportunities to volunteer or contribute, and a shared sense of community and responsibility, is to reverse the current trend for service providers to grow, merge and take each other over and instead scale down. Small organisations can achieve the behaviours and feel of mutual ownership more easily than large ones. Very small community groups and enterprises could not feasibly form Industrial Provident Societies and other legal forms of cooperative, and may even be effectively private sector, but nevertheless can have a more mutual 'feel' to them than a large NHS Foundation Trust, because of the kinds of relationships within them.

I have outlined how personal budgets could be an opportunity for people to form small groups around shared needs, goals and responsibilities, if personal-budget holders were more able to find and network with each other, and front-line workers. So one version of a mutual future for public services would be the combination of individual control over resources, coupled with the social media infrastructure and human support to connect with each other and with local providers, both established and start-up.

Additionally, it would be possible to reform the whole concept of the personal budget, from being purely an amount of money to spend on a service, to being an ownership stake in a service. While offering cooperative-style shared ownership to their users would not be attractive to private-sector providers (although legislation could mandate this where a private organisation collapses or repeatedly fails inspections), it would offer a way for public sector providers and charities to reform along mutual lines.

Many charities and housing associations have grown from their roots as small groups established by concerned citizens into multimillion-pound service contractors, which can feel distant to their 'beneficiaries' and volunteers, who have more access to or control over their boards than they do over public and private-sector organisations. These mega-charities could consider whether the charitable trust model still connects them to the people who founded them, or if they would be better handing their services back to local people to control in the form of a franchise, while retaining a smaller central charity to support their work and provide national campaigning and fundraising capacity.

Regulating the new system

In Chapter Three I outlined the limitations in regulation and inspections in keeping people safe. The premise for the existence of a regulator is deficit-based: an independent body with statutory powers is needed to find those public services that are failing, or even dangerous, and to protect vulnerable people using those services who couldn't otherwise protect themselves. What would regulation look like if it was fully aligned with an asset-based public service system whose overarching role was to promote and maintain wellbeing?

Regulation would retain its focus on its role in keeping people safe and identifying when a public service is not safe, because there always will be failing organisations in most public service sectors and without safety there can be no wellbeing. Regulators, though, would see safety in the context of overall wellbeing.

Currently, quality is perhaps the word that service providers and commissioners use most often when talking about the value of what they do. A good-quality service recruits using sound recruitment processes, has clear policies and procedures in place and keeps clear records of what it does. These are all good things and their absence tends to indicate that a service does not do a consistently good job, but when applied to long-term support services, they do not on their own amount to a service that supports good lives. Quality does not describe the outcomes, experiences, rights and relationships of people using a service. When a service focuses exclusively on quality, it is likely to be rooted in the belief that it and its workers can fix people's problems, providing they are well-organised enough. It is likely to find the messiness of ordinary life problematic.

So regulators need to ensure that public services have the systems in place that add up to quality, but they need to put that achievement of quality in the wider context of how people live their lives. So Shared Lives schemes are inspected by CQC on their quality and safety, but this is done in the context of a service that is expected to be good at helping Shared Lives households to build and live ordinary lives. This is an approach to regulation that sees the systems and policies of a service as the foundations and walls of a sound house, but the value of the house to those living in it is the extent to which it feels like home.

An asset-based approach to regulation would see a service as having a vital role to play in safety, but would be suspicious of models in which the service was seen as having the sole responsibility for that. Shared Lives is consistently rated by inspectors as the highest performing kind of care partly because people living in and visiting Shared Lives households are typically visible members of their community with lots of friends who would raise concerns if they had them. Contrast this with a large care home where staff rotas preclude people from spending time in the community and everyone who has contact with the residents is either an employee of the service or one of its volunteers.

Data collection and sharing has a role to play in this model of regulation, because it is another way to set the quality of systems and practices in the context the results they achieve. Clearly this is only helpful if the data collected gives a full picture of people's wellbeing and their experience of a service, rather than recording only process or a narrow range of physical health outcomes. It would be important to share this data with the people who used the service and their families, giving them the opportunity to use it to suggest changes and improvements.

An asset-based regulator would recognise that only the people and families using a service themselves can complete an accurate picture of the effectiveness of a service, so it would invest a significant proportion of its resources in supporting people to share their experiences and would expect every service to have structures that enabled people to talk with each other about what was working and what was not, with records of actions taken as a result. This would include consultative committees of the kind that many services already have in place, but would also need to include a range of options for people to share their views confidently and safely. Inspectors would employ a much greater number of people with first-hand experience of using the relevant services as part of refocusing inspection on what matters most and ensuring that some 'patients' or 'service users' were regarded as 'colleagues' and 'inspectors'.

Integrating the new system

This book aims to set out a new model for long-term support. It focuses most heavily on the kinds of long-term support that impact on nearly all of us during our lifetimes: health and social care. But, as in the example given earlier of aligning the system around the emotional and financial stability of families, for the new system to be given the most chance of success, we would have to be prepared to go further than this, into areas of the state such as housing and welfare benefits, which are most resistant to radical change and where seeing people first and foremost as people with capacity and potential is least in evidence.

There have been attempts to introduce personal budgets into welfare-to-work programmes, which, despite their apparent success, were quietly shelved due to their lack of fit with a political narrative that was increasingly punitive. There is a strong argument for seeing people who are seeking work as having capacity and potential: few of us successfully win a job when we lack confidence in our abilities. But it is difficult to introduce asset-based thinking into a sector that is more concerned with being seen to manage the phantoms of 'scroungers' and benefits fraud.

There have even been small-scale attempts to offer personal budgets and other responsibility-sharing approaches to offenders. Offenders are typically seen as the least trustworthy and least deserving groups of people supported by the state, yet the primary goal in supporting them is to see them become responsible citizens again, which can only happen if they and those around them can recognise and build their potential.

The model set out would be an integrated service model. Integrating services, particularly integrating different parts of the NHS and integrating the NHS with social care is something of a holy grail for service planners. There have been plans to achieve it produced at least annually almost from the birth of the NHS. By integration, people usually mean either merged, joined-up or just better-aligned public service organisations. By establishing a single, shared set of goals – wellbeing – for all long-term support services, we would achieve a much deeper and more desirable form of integration. At present, the most likely outcome of health and social care integration would be services being merged into the power base of the local hospital trust: a decisive move away from communities and towards the needs of the most medical and institutional model of care. Unifying our services around a set of human goals would be a move in the opposite direction. With a range of services working towards the same goal, resource sharing and formal integration would follow in some cases, perhaps even at central government level where a single department for public services would make more sense than the territorial and competing departments that each manage a part of our health, council, offender management, back-to-work and social care services.

The importance of scaling down, closing things and letting go

A common challenge to those working in and supporting small, human-scale interventions and social enterprises is, 'That's lovely. But how are you going to scale it up?' An equally valid challenge to those running large institutions and bureaucracies is: how are you going to scale down?

Before resources can be found to scale up interventions that are a good fit for people's lives, those resources must be liberated from our largest institutions. In business, from where much recent public service culture has been derived, the goal is growth, but growth cannot be an end in itself for public services. Those working on a large scale, who challenge small initiatives to scale up, should perhaps reflect on the fact that even a tiny initiative, which is successfully collaborating with people and their networks to help them live well, is already successful, whereas an organisation that has grown distant and disconnected from people and human-sized goals is failing, and failing big. When toxic, one-way, inflexible relationships between people and systems are spread on a larger and larger scale this is not success: it's a tumour.

Inspection results consistently correlate better support with smaller services. There are of course exceptions to that rule: large organisations that work hard to stay locally rooted and to devolve decision-making and relationship-building power down to the front line. They often have branch or franchise structures and they focus on adding backup and resources without stifling creativity and autonomy. But there are others that have confused growth – and the accompanying trappings of large salaries, big offices and leverage with government – with success. It is unlikely that these services will scale down without legislation forcibly transferring power from them to the people who currently use them.

One way to tackle the entrenchment of large services, particularly those that occupy large buildings, is to recognise that those buildings and the services within them are two separate things. Buildings that people live in or visit regularly for a long time also contain relationships; sometimes those people's most important relationships. That different view opens up the possibility of considering what would be the best use and design of those three kinds of asset.

This would help to separate genuine attempts to improve people's lives through new kinds of support, from closures that (despite the inevitable use of terms like 'modernisation') are thoughtless cost-cutting exercises. It would enable a different kind of conversation about the future of services like day centres, which can often become an ideological battleground. One side believes that day centres embody segregation and institutionalisation. The other side believes that the alternative to day centres is casting disabled or older people out into a solitary existence in a 'community' that turns out to be at best elusive, and at worst, openly hostile.

Destructive debates about building-based services could often be avoided if, instead of asking 'Should this service close?', decision makers asked:

1 How could this building best be used, and by whom?
2 What support do people want; how and where is that support best delivered?
3 What relationships are there between the people who use this building, and how could those relationships continue, or be replaced by new ones, as people wish?

So the building could continue to be used by some of the current groups, but also made available to others within the local community (this could mean it was used for more of the day and became more cost-effective too). Some of the services could continue, others could end and new ones could begin; some carrying on within the building and some in new locations. And fewer people with learning disabilities would find themselves hanging around the local shopping centre, personal assistant in tow, bored and lonely.

Even in hospitals, there have been attempts to think more clearly about the difference between the building full of beds and machines, and the people and services the building houses. 'Virtual wards' for older people at high risk of hospitalisation, but whose ongoing treatment and monitoring was not reliant on a hospital environment, involved those people receiving care from hospital staff and others at home, with support to self-care as far as possible. At a hospital, practitioners need only walk from bed to bed rather than travelling from house to house, so their time is used efficiently, but the downside is the expense of maintaining the hotel function of a hospital, plus the considerable health risks and loss of independence of being in hospital for an extended period. Virtual wards enabled people to stay well and at home, although realising any tangible savings to the NHS to offset the additional costs proved harder (Lewis et al, 2013).

The only way that moving care out of hospital would save real money is if an entire ward, or entire hospital could be closed. There is an argument in some areas (particularly densely populated urban areas with several hospitals) for the deeply unpopular idea of merging some services and closing some buildings. But in most cases, the bar of creating real savings, from hospital closures, is unrealistically high: used as a reason not to make changes that cannot hope to reach it. It also no longer reflects the large and growing gap between those services that are needed and those that remain uncut, with spiralling waiting lists for procedures that can only be carried out in hospital. If the three questions given earlier were asked of hospitals, we would conclude that some of the services would be best placed elsewhere, but that the buildings were still needed. The transition needed is not to a world where people have to wait ever longer for an operation, or travel further in an emergency, but to hospitals becoming the supportive partner to the main focus of community-based healthcare and, perhaps, in which the NHS itself is willing to play a supporting role to social and community care, where the biggest wellbeing gains are to be found.

Escaping the invisible asylum: actions

1. Plan slowly to move fast

Most public services work like this: assess, plan, support, review. It doesn't work. Instead, offer just enough support, while planning, and review that plan constantly. If plans are portable (this can simply mean they given to the person on a piece of paper), there is more opportunity for the services they come into contact with to build up a picture of the whole person over time, rather than just a snapshot of a crisis. A plan can only be portable (intelligible and relevant to any public service worker who reads it) if all public services share the same goal of wellbeing.

2. Open the floodgates

For a long time, the expert view of flood control was based on building walls. The higher the wall, the safer the community behind it. Now the opposite view has taken hold: share some land with the rivers and sea, creating environments that can survive inundation and thrive on its natural cycle. Services are necessary, but not what people dream of or covet, unless they are desperate and there is nothing else. We need to open the gates, go outside and seek people as early as we can find them. If we have time to understand what they really want and need in life, our services will be a vital – but small – part of it.

3. Combine our assets

The choice we face is not between professional services and volunteers. We need to be able to combine formal and informal, paid and unpaid contributions. We need access to expertise, but to value the insight that only an individual, family or community can have into their own capabilities. Shared Lives carers continually demonstrates that there is little we cannot achieve when we do this.

4. Stop magical thinking and hero worship

We all need to recognise that while our public services and the people who work in them are a vital part of a civilised society and have achieved many things, they cannot fix us or our communities. Only we can do that. If we are more realistic about the things that iconic figures like the NHS family doctor cannot do for us, we may also be more appreciative of what they can do, as well as what we need to do for ourselves to live well.

5. The services we need already exist

There are already enough cost-effective interventions on which to build a new system. Those in charge of public service budgets need to get serious in investing in them, or find ways of giving control of that money to people, including people who use services and their families, who will.

6. The future is mutual

The customer service model of long-term support services never works. It is riddled with lies and ways to infantilise 'customers'. If a service means it when it says everything it does revolves around the people it serves, then some of them will be in paid roles in those organisations and all of them will be its co-owners.

7. Measure your harm

Every public service inadvertently causes at least some harm. That does not make public services bad or wrong: it just means they are not powered by magic. Being prepared to cause harm, like being prepared to take risks, is essential to public services being willing and able to intervene in people's lives. At present, public services continue to feel able to intervene in our lives through pretending they do no harm. This removes the possibility of reducing that harm, or deciding not to intervene when the likely harm outweighs the possible gains. We must measure that harm and weigh it up against the good: the balance will be the wellbeing we have created.

8. Fund public services adequately

Nothing in this book happens free of charge. The changes in it will only improve public services if we invest a realistic level of GDP in them.

Can we escape?

Every sanctuary has the potential to become prison-like, and it is hard to escape from a prison you cannot see, or refuse to see. I have never been in doubt of the achievements of our public services. Those achievements are often miraculous, if frequently unnoticed, whereas the problems are deep-rooted, contestable and constantly spun into political yarns. Start looking closely at health and care services and you are quickly tangled up in byzantine service structures, jargon and acronyms. But the arcana obscures some simple divisions which were built into our concept of support from the beginning: who is a citizen and who is a ward of the state; those who need fixing and those who fix. As we live longer, but spend longer within service systems, we will all find ourselves on the wrong side of those divisions, where 'home' becomes 'care home', everyday choices become risks to assess, and the gap between the life we are living and want to live becomes 'presenting need'.

Those of us involved in public services in some way, whether as people who use support, family carers, front-line workers or managers and leaders, face a corrosive choice: ignore those divides and the dissonance they create or rail ineffectually against them.

The gains of social care's 'personalisation' hint at the value of scaling things down to the individual level, and also the limitations of our power to effect change as unconnected individuals. The quiet, slow and patchy growth of Shared Lives demonstrates the power of joining back together, not to form new bureaucracies, but into new kinds of household, community and even national movements.

If we escape the invisible asylum rather than continually patching it up, our crumbling services will not just be more saveable, we will feel more passionate about saving them. Even more remarkable than the technological or medical miracles are the unnoticed miracles of caring that thousands of underpaid or unpaid people achieve every day, within systems they cannot fully see or comprehend, but whose crushing embrace they feel all too well. That instinct to care for one another is the beginning of everything good that happens within our public services; we imprison it at our peril.

Notes

Chapter One

1. www.my-life.org.uk. Quotation from: www.in-control.org.uk/support/support-for-individuals,-family-members-carers/personal-stories/caroline-tomlinson.aspx.

2. 'Social prescribing' is an example of an attempt to change this, through enabling GPs to 'prescribe' a social intervention (such as a support group or fitness activity), for problems which lack a medical cause.

3. *The Care Act 2014* avoided moving to a so-called 'carer-blind' eligibility system, in which support was offered regardless of the level of family care available. In countries with 'carer-blind' assessment systems, individuals have a choice as to whether to seek their support from the state or from their family.

4. MRSA and other drug-resistant bugs were for a time a health-service bogeyman, killing many older people in hospital and causing widespread fear until the bugs were much reduced, not by new drugs or technology, but simply by staff getting better at washing their hands.

5. This risk is shockingly high for people in their 80s. A typical woman aged 85 uses 100% of her quadriceps muscle power to stand up unaided and loses 5% of that muscle power after 12 hours in a hospital bed. In other words, a single day in hospital can be enough to render the older person unable to live independently, without intensive physiotherapy to regain the strength to do so.

6. I am indebted to Liz Sargeant, an expert in hospital discharge and many other things, for this phrase.

7. Offenders who have housing issues after custody are more likely to reoffend and addressing accommodation is a 'necessary if not sufficient' for reducing reoffending (Ministry of Justice, 2014; Maguire and Nolan, 2007).

8. There are limits to this inclusivity, particularly for disabled parents who find the school run physically inaccessible.

9. Michael Brown OBE, a police inspector who tweets as @mentalhealthcop, gives ongoing insight into the experience of attempting to provide compassionate and effective responses to people with mental health problems, from within a police service poorly resourced and trained to do so.

Chapter Two

1. 'Dementia care: your stories', *BBC News*, 18 May 2012. Available at: www.bbc.co.uk/news/health-18116016.
2. 'Home care workers "not properly vetted"', *BBC News*, 15 October 2012. Available at: www.bbc.co.uk/news/health-19944217; BBC TV *Inside Out* programme broadcast 19 October 2012.
3. BBC Radio 4 File on 4, 28 February 2017.
4. Nicholson ran the body with responsibility for oversight of Mid Staffordshire and other organisations. A sustained *Daily Mail* hate campaign dubbed him 'the man with no shame' until he left this job.
5. I co-chaired this group alongside a civil servant.

Chapter Three

1. Tom Bennett, government appointed head of a task force to improve teacher training in England, quoted in *The Guardian* in 2015. Available at: www.theguardian.com/education/2015/jun/16/schools-ignore-bad-behaviour-fool-ofsted-tom-bennett.

Chapter Four

1. Personally, I would query whether 'learned' or 'over' dependence is always the failure or negative outcome it is seen to be. It can be risky or harmful to develop a close relationship with a staff member who in all likelihood will move on, or which exacerbates the power imbalances within large services. But nearly all of us want and need to feel dependent on someone: 'inappropriate' emotional dependence reflects the limitations of the relationships possible within certain kinds of service, not necessarily of the people involved.
2. The notional cost of not taking an opportunity to create an improvement or benefit to someone's health or wellbeing.
3. See the work of Dr Jenny Morris OBE, Michelle Wates, the Disabled Parents Network and The Carers' Trust.
4. This is of course a mainstream Western account in which success is correlated with financial independence and economic mobility, rather than

with maintaining a cohesive extended family. Housing price rises and other pressures are making shared housing and 'boomerang kids' more common, and the life course described increasingly delayed or unaffordable, although it remains the goal for most.

Chapter Five

1. The National Audit Office found that the evidence of impact for personal budgets was weak and drew from this broad conclusions about the progress of personalisation, in a report which used those terms interchangeably (Burkett et al, 2016).
2. http://sharedlivesplus.org.uk/news/staff-blog/item/232-A%20leap%20 in%20the%20dark.
3. As cited in the NHS England Excellence in Participation Awards 2014.
4. Big Society was a policy initiative championed and later abandoned by Prime Minister David Cameron's Conservative government.
5. Small Good Stuff: www.smallgoodstuff.co.uk.

Chapter Six

1. Alison's and Chris's quotes come from an entry written by Birmingham Shared Lives scheme for the author's blog in 2016.
2. Unpublished national safeguarding data, shared with the author in 2016.

Chapter Seven

1. I'm grateful to Dame Philippa Russell for this observation.
2. Health Secretary Jeremy Hunt, for instance, in a 2013 speech to social care leaders, said the UK should adopt 'Asian attitudes' to caring for parents.
3. I'm using 'family' in its broadest sense: the people with whom we form a household.
4. There are various similar definitions of 'co-production'. See Think Local, Act Personal's National Co-production Advisory Group. Available at: https://www.thinklocalactpersonal.org.uk/co-production-in-commissioning-tool/.

Chapter Eight

1. Unpublished case study supplied by LAC Network, 2017.
2. Hyatt was speaking at People Powered Health, an event hosted by Nesta, May 2017.
3. Presentation to the King's Fund, 12 July 2016.

References

Age UK (2017) *Briefing: Health and Care of Older People in England 2017*, London: Age UK.

Aldridge, J. and Becker, S. (2003) *Children Caring for Parents With Mental Illness: Perspectives of Young Carers, Parents and Professionals*, Oxford: Blackwell Science.

Aldridge, J., Becker, S. and Dearden, C. (1998) *Young Carers and Their Families*, Oxford: Blackwell Science.

Autism Together (2015) *Mate Crime in Merseyside*, Wirral: Wirral Autistic Society.

Bate, P. (2005) *In Praise of Slow Inclusion*, Bath: National Development Team.

Bennett, S. (2014) *Getting Serious About Personalisation in the NHS*, London: Think Local, Act Personal.

Blood, I. (2013) *A Better Life: Valuing Our Later Years*, York: Joseph Rowntree Foundation.

Bloodworth, J. (2017) 'All the horror stories I came across as a care worker were about employers', *The Guardian*, 20 February 2017. Available at: www.theguardian.com/commentisfree/2017/feb/20/horror-stories-care-worker-employers-care-slots-five-minutes.

Bolton, J. (2016) *Predicting and Managing Demand in Social Care*, discussion paper, Oxford: Oxford Brookes University, Institute of Public Care.

Bowers, H. (2009) *Older People's Vision for Long Term Care*, York: Joseph Rowntree Foundation.

Bowers, H., Lockwood, S., Eley, A., Catley, A., Runnicles, D., Mordey, M., Barker, S., Thomas, N., Jones, C. and Dalziel, D. (2013) *Widening Choices for Older People With High Support Needs*, York: Joseph Rowntree Foundation.

Bowers, H., Mordey, M., Runnicles, D., Barker, S., Thomas, N., Wilkins, A., National Development Team for Inclusion, Lockwood, S., Catley, A., and Community Catalysts (2011) *JRF Programme Paper, Better Life: Not a One Way Street – Research Into Older People's Experiences of Support Based on Mutuality and Reciprocity, Interim Findings*, October, York: Joseph Rowntree Foundation.

Boyles, J. (ed.) (2017) *Psychological Therapies for Survivors of Torture*, Monmouth: PCCS Books.

Brindle, D. (2008) 'Tireless Champion of Autonomy', *The Guardian*, 22 October. Available at: www.theguardian.com/society/2008/oct/21/john-evans.

Broad, R. (2015) *People, Places, Possibilities*, Sheffield: The Centre for Welfare Reform.

Brunton, D. (2004) *Medicine Transformed: Health, Disease & Society in Europe, 1800-1930*, Manchester: The Open University.

Buckner, L. and Yeandle, S. (2015) *Valuing Carers 2015: The Rising Value of Carers' Support*, London: Carers UK.

Burd, H. and Hallsworth, M. (2016) *Supporting Self-Management: A Guide to Enabling Behaviour Change for Health and Wellbeing Using Person- and Community-Centred Approaches*, London: Nesta and The Behavioural Insights Team.

Burkett, M., Dina, A., King, J., Martin, R., Barreto, O.P., Quick, H., Whittingham, A. and Woolley, C. (2016) *Personalised Commissioning in Adult Social Care*, London: National Audit Office.

Cahn, E. and Rowe, J. (1992) *Time Dollars: The New Currency that Enables Americans to Turn Their Hidden Resource - Time - into Personal Security & Community Renewal*, Emmaus, Pennsylvania: Rodale.

Callan, S. (2011) *Completing the Revolution: Transforming Mental Health and Tackling Poverty*, London: Centre for Social Justice.

Carson, G. (2017) 'Man with learning disabilities wins damages after human rights breach', *Community Care*, 17 August. Available at: www.communitycare.co.uk/2017/08/17/man-learning-disabilities-wins-damages-human-rights-breach.

Carter, R. (2016) 'Care cuts: "If it meets needs and costs less then we have no choice"', *Community Care*, 8 August. Available at: www.communitycare.co.uk/2016/08/03/meets-needs-costs-less-dont-choice-impact-cuts-personalisation/.

Chanan, G. (ed.) (2011) *Empowering Communities for Health Business Case and Practice Framework*, Exeter: NHS Alliance.

Clarence, E. and Gabriel, M. (2014) *People Helping People: The Future of Public Services*, London: Nesta.

CLG (Communities and Local Government Committee) (2017) *Adult Social Care Inquiry*, London: HMSO.

CMA (Competitions and Market Authority) (2017) Care Homes Market Study Update Paper, London: CMA.

Cooke, G. and Muir, R. (eds) (2012) *The Relational State*, London: ippr.

Co-operative College and Change AGEnts (2017) *Owning Our Care: Investigating the Development of Multi-Stakeholder Co-operative Social Care in the UK*, Manchester: Co-operative College and Change AGEnts.

CQC (Care Quality Commission) (2017) *The State of Adult Social Care in England 2014 to 2017*, London: CQC.

CQC (Care Quality Commission) (2016) *Right Here, Right Now*, London: CQC.

CQC (Care Quality Commission) (2012) *Learning Disability Services Inspection Programme: National Overview*, London: Care Quality Commission.

Davidson, S. and Rossall, P. (2014) *Evidence Review: Loneliness in Later Life*, London: Age UK.

Del Castillo, J., Khan, H., Nicholas, L. and Finnis, A. (2016) *Health as a Social Movement: The Power of People in Movements*, London: Nesta.

Department for Work and Pensions (2013) *Fulfilling Potential: Making It Happen for Disabled People*, London: Office for Disability Issues and DWP.

Department of Health (2012) *Long-Term Conditions Compendium of Information* (3rd edn), London: HMSO.

Dewing, J. and McCormack, B. (2016) 'Tell me, how do you define person-centredness?' *Journal of Clinical Nursing*, 26(17/18): 2509-10. Available at: http://onlinelibrary.wiley.com/doi/10.1111/jocn.13681/pdf.

EHRC (Equality and Human Rights Commission) (2011) *Close to Home: An Inquiry Into Older People and Human Rights in Home Care*, London: EHRC.

Foot, J. (2016) *The Man Who Closed the Asylums*, London: Verso.

Forder, J., Jones, K., Glendinning, C., Caiels, J., Welch, E., Baxter, K., Davidson, J., Windle, K., Irvine, A., King, D. and Dolan, P. (2012) *Personal Health Budgets Pilot Evaluation*, London: Personal Health Budgets Evaluation Partnership.

Fox, A. (2015) 'Growing up Sharing My Life', in author's blog, 12 January. Available at: https://alexfoxblog.wordpress.com/2015/01/12/growing-up-sharing-my-life/.

Fox, A., Lockwood, S., Stansfield, J., Waters, J. and Broad, R. (2013) *Redesigning the Front End of Social Care*, np: In Control, Community Catalysts, Shared Lives Plus and Inclusive Neighbourhoods. Available at: http://sharedlivesplus.org.uk/images/publications/Redesigning_the_front_end_of_social_care_final.pdf.

Francis, R. (2013) *Report of the Mid Staffordshire NHS Foundation Trust Public Inquiry*, London: The Stationery Office.

Giddens, A. (1998) *The Third Way: The Renewal of Social Democracy*, Cambridge: Polity Press.

Gilburt, H. (2015) *Mental Health Under Pressure*, London: The King's Fund.

Goffman, G. (1961) *Asylums*, London: Penguin.

Greenstreet, R. (2011) 'I didn't want them to take my baby', *The Guardian*, 21 July. Available at: www.theguardian.com/lifeandstyle/2012/jul/21/shared-lives-caring-scheme.

Hall, K., Needham, C. and Allen, K. (2014) 'Grass roots entrepreneurship and innovation: micro-enterprises in social care'. Paper for International Research Society for Public Management Annual Conference, Ottawa, Canada, April.

Halpern, D. (2010) *The Hidden Wealth of Nations*, Cambridge: Polity Press.

Hattenstone, S. (2016) '"We never thought he wouldn't come home": Why did our son, Connor Sparrowhawk, die?' *The Guardian*, 2 April. Available at: www.theguardian.com/society/2016/apr/02/never-thought-he-wouldnt-come-home-why-son-connor-sparrowhawk-die.

Hatton, C. and Waters, J. (2014) *Third National Personal Budgets Survey*, London: Think Local Act Personal, In Control and Lancaster University.

Hayek, F. (1945) 'The use of knowledge in society', *American Economic Review*, 35(4): 519-30.

Health Care Leader (2015) 'Three care homes now rated outstanding by CQC', *Health Care Leader*, 19 May. Available at: http://healthcareleadernews.com/article/three-care-homes-now-rated-outstanding-cqc.

Healthwatch England (2017) *Home Care Services: What People Told Healthwatch About Their Experiences*, Newcastle: Healthwatch England.

Hills, J. (2014) *Good Times, Bad Times: The Welfare Myth of Them and Us*, Bristol: Policy Press.

HM Government (2007) *Putting People First: A Shared Vision and Commitment to the Transformation of Adult Social Care*, London: HM Government.

Hofmann, S., Asnaani, A., Vonk, I.J.J., Sawyer, A.T. and Fang, A. (2012) 'The efficacy of cognitive behavioral therapy: A review of meta-analyses', *Cognitive Therapy and Research*, 36(5): 427-40.

Holt-Lunstad, J., Smith, T.B. and Layton, J.B. (2010) 'Social relationships and mortality risk: A meta-analytic review', *PLoS Medicine*, 7(7). Available at: http://journals.plos.org/plosmedicine/article?id=10.1371/journal.pmed.1000316.

Honoré, C. (2005) *In Praise of Slowness*, San Francisco: Harper.

Illich, I. (1974) *Medical Nemesis: The Expropriation of Health*, London: Calder & Boyars.

Kempton, J. and Tomlin, S. (2014) *Ageing Alone: Loneliness and the 'Oldest Old'*, London: CentreForum.

Knapp, M., Bauer, A., Perkins, M. and Snell, T. (2011) *Building Community Capacity: Making an Economic Case*. PSSRU Discussion Paper 2772, London: Personal Social Services Research Unit, LSE.

Kretzmann, J.P. and McKnight, J.L. (1993) *Building Communities From the Inside Out: A Path Toward Finding and Mobilizing a Community's Assets*, Evanston, IL: Institute for Policy Research.

Leadbeater, C. (2004) *Personalisation through Participation: A New Script for Public Services*, London: Demos.

Learning Disabilities Observatory (2016) *People With Learning Disabilities in England 2015: Main Report*, London: Public Health England.

Lessof, C., Ross, A., Brind, R., Bell, E. and Newton, S. (2016) *Longitudinal Study of Young People in England, Cohort 2: Health and Wellbeing at Wave 2*, London: Department for Education.

Lewis, F. (2015) *Estimation of Future Cases of Dementia From Those Born in 2015*, London: Alzheimer's Research UK.

Lewis, G., Vaithianathan, R., Wright, L. and Bardsley, M. (2013) 'Integrating care for high-risk patients in England using the virtual ward model: lessons in the process of care integration from three case sites', *International Journal of Integrated Care*, 13(4): e046.

MacInnes, T., Tinson, A., Hughes, C., Born, T.B. and Aldridge, H. (2015) *Monitoring Poverty and Social Exclusion 2015*, York: Joseph Rowntree Foundation.

Maguire, M. and Nolan, J. (2007) 'Accommodation and related services for ex-prisoners', in A. Hucklesby and L. Hagley-Dickinson (eds) *Prisoner Resettlement: Policy and Practice*, Devon: Willan.

Marcus, G., Neumark, T. and Broome, S. (2011) *Power Lines*, London: RSA.

Mason, M. (2012) *Care Home Sweet Home: Care Home of the Future*, London: International Longevity Centre UK.

McKnight, J. (1995) *The Careless Society: Community and Its Counterfeits*, Chicago, IL: Basic Books.

McShane, M. and Mitchell, E. (2013) 'Integrating care for people with comorbidities', *HSJ*, 9 July. Available at: www.hsj.co.uk/sectors/commissioning/integrating-care-for-people-with-comorbidities/5060119.article.

Ministry of Justice (2014) *Transforming Rehabilitation: A Summary of Evidence on Reducing Reoffending* (2nd edn), London: Ministry of Justice Analytical Series.

Moriarty, J. (2014) *Personalisation for People From Black and Minority Ethnic Groups*, London: Race Equality Foundation.

Mount, B. (1992) *Person Centred Planning: A Sourcebook of Values, Ideas and Methods to Encourage Person-Centered Development*, New York: Graphic Futures.

Mulgan, G. (2010) *The Birth of the Relational State*, London: ippr.

Munro, E., Hollingworth, K., Meetoo, V., Quy, K., McDermid, S., Trivedi, H. and Holmes, L. (2014) *Residential Parenting Assessments: Uses, Costs and Contributions to Effective and Timely Decision-Making in Public Law Cases*, research report, July, London: DfE.

Naylor, C., Mundle, C., Weaks, L. and Buck, D. (2013) *Volunteering in Health and Care: Securing a Sustainable Future*, London: King's Fund.

Neary, M. (2014) 'The personal budget review', Love, Belief and Balls blog, 17 May. Available at: https://markneary1dotcom1. wordpress.com/2014/05/27/the-personal-budget-review/.

Needham, C. and Carr, S. (2015) 'Micro-provision of social care support for marginalized communities – filling the gap or building bridges to the mainstream?' *Social Policy & Administration*, 49(7): 824-41.

Needham, C. and Glasby, J. (eds) (2014) *Debates in Personalisation*, Bristol: Policy Press.

NHS Digital (2016) *Personal Social Services Adult Social Care Survey England 2015-16*, Leeds: NHS Digital.

NHS Digital (2014) *Adult Social Care Outcomes Framework Data*, London: Health and Social Care Information Centre.

Norcross, J. (2011) *Evidence-Based Therapy Relationships Task Force Conclusions*, New York: The Society for the Advancement of Psychotherapy.

O'Brien, J. (2015) *Surviving Cogworld? Supporting People With Disabilities in a Mechanistic System*, Madison, WI: Developmental Disabilities Network.

O'Brien, J. (1989) *What's Worth Working For? Leadership for Better Quality Human Services*, Lithonia, GA: Responsive Systems Associates.

O'Brien, J. and O'Brien, C.L. (1988) *A Little Book About Person Centred Planning*, Toronto: Inclusion Press.

Oliver, M., Sapey, B. and Thomas, P. (1983) *Social Work With Disabled People*, London: Palgrave Macmillan.

Parsfield, M. (ed.) (2015) *Community Capital: The Value of Connected Communities*, London: RSA.

Porter, R. (2006) *Madmen: A Social History of Madhouses, Mad-Doctors & Lunatics*, Stroud: Tempus.

RCN (Royal College of Nursing) (2015) *Briefing: The Buurtzorg Nederland (Home Care Provider) Model: Observations for the UK*, London: RCN, updated 2016. Available at: www.rcn.org.uk/about-us/policy-briefings/br-0215.

Rothwell, J. (director) (2008) *Heavy Load* (documentary film).

Rowson, J., Broome, S. and Jones, A. (2010) *Connected Communities: How Social Networks Power and Sustain the Big Society*, London: RSA.

Ryan, S. (2017) '"I want to ask you a little about your blog…"', My Daft Life blog, 12 August. Available at: https://mydaftlife.com.

Ryan, S. (2014) 'Background briefing on mother's blog', Entry to My Daft Life blog, 8 October. Available at: https://mydaftlife.com.

Shared Lives Plus (2017) *The State of Shared Lives in England*, Liverpool: Shared Lives Plus.

Shared Lives Plus (2015) *A Shared Life Is a Healthy Life*, Liverpool: Shared Lives Plus.

Sheffield, H. (2017) 'Why co-operatives could be the answer to the UK's social care crisis', *The Independent*, 1 August. Available at: www.independent.co.uk/news/business/indyventure/social-care-co-op-uk-crisis-entrepreneur-age-careshare-labour-a7862611.html.

Siddique, H. (2016) 'Under-fire Southern Health chief resigns over "media attention"', *The Guardian*, 30 August. Available at: https://www.theguardian.com/society/2016/aug/30/southern-health-chief-quits-connor-sparrowhawk-death.

Sitch, T. (ed.) (2014) *Thurrock Local Area Coordination: Fourteen Month Evaluation Report*, Thurrock: Thurrock Council.

Skills for Care (2012) *The State of the Adult Social Care Sector and Workforce in England 2012*, London: Skills for Care.

Smith, D. (2016) 'The outstanding Yorkshire care home: "We aim to give people the care we'd want"', *The Guardian*, 1 March. Available at: www.theguardian.com/social-care-network/2016/mar/01/outstanding-care-home-cqc-older-people.

Social Exclusion Unit (2002) *Reducing Re-offending by Ex-Prisoners*, London: SEU.

TLAP (Think Local Act Personal), National Voices and NHS England (2014) *No Assumptions: A Narrative for Personalised, Coordinated Care and Support in Mental Health*, London: Think Local Act Personal and National Voices.

Todd, R. and Williams, B. (2013) *Investing in Shared Lives*, London: Social Finance.

Turner, A. (2017) 'CQC relaxes stance on "bed limit" for learning disability services', *Community Care*, 13 June. Available at: www.communitycare.co.uk/2017/06/13/cqc-relaxes-stance-bed-limit-learning-disability-services/.

UKHCA (United Kingdom Homecare Association) (2012) *Care Is Not a Commodity*, London: UKHCA.

Vanier, J. (1979) *Community and Growth*, London: Longman.

Waddell, G. and Burton, A.K. (2006) *Is Work Good for Your Health and Well-Being?* London: The Stationery Office.

Walker, P. (2011a) 'Gemma Hayter case review finds chances were missed to protect her', *The Guardian*, 14 November. Available at: www.theguardian.com/society/2011/nov/14/gemma-hayter-case-review.

Walker, P. (2011b) 'Police are failing people with learning disabilities, says study', *The Guardian*, 20 June. Available at: www.theguardian.com/society/2011/jun/20/police-failing-learning-disabilities-study.

Wates, M. (2002) *Supporting Disabled Adults in Their Parenting Role*, York: Joseph Rowntree Foundation.

Welch, E., Caiels, J., Bass, R., Jones, K., Forder, J. and Windle, K. (2013) *Implementing Personal Health Budgets Within Substance Misuse Services*, PSSRU Discussion Paper 2858, Canterbury: Kent University.

Wood, S., Finnis, A., Khan, H., Ejbye, J. (2016) *Realising the Value of People and Communities*, London: Health Foundation and Nesta.

WTPN (Working Together With Parents Network) (2016) *Working Together With Parents Network (WTPN): Update of the DoH/DfES Good Practice Guidance on Working With Parents With a Learning Disability*, Bristol: University of Bristol.

Index

reciprocity 82, 131, 139, 157, 195, 200, 207
records, ownership of 183
reductionist approach 47
regulation 48, 49, 50–3, 71, 159, 209–11
relapsing/remitting health conditions 18
'relational state' 7
Remploy 53
research 54–8, 78–9, 202–3
research and development (R&D) approach 202
resilience-building
  as aim 141, 145, 148, 154–5, 183
  funding for 205, 206
  Local Area Coordination 184
  measurement of 146
  relationships and 43, 44, 50, 157, 176
'Resource Allocation Systems' 93
responsibility of citizenship 5, 26, 81–4, 163, 164
responsibility, shared 163–5
'reverse auctions' 37
Revolving Doors 19
the right
  and market forces 6
  on responsibility 83
risk 69–85
  aversion 75–7
  and citizenship 73
  and hospital 17
  organisational 75–6
  and responsibility 81–4
risky behaviours 74, 149
Robin Lane Practice, Leeds 193
Roper, Adrian 207
Royal Society of Arts (RSA) 144, 171, 179

S

Salford Dadz 180
Sanderson, Helen 191
scaling down 212–15
'sectioning' 98
self-advocacy organisations *see* user-led organisations

'self-care' 164
Self-Directed Support 88, 89
self-employment 195–8
Shared Lives 8–10, 109–41, 163–4, 181, 201
  Care Quality Commission and 111, 129, 196, 210
  connections 157
  costs 118, 119
  ethos 140–1
  and fluctuating support needs 18
  friendship 115, 116
  independence and interdependence 122–6
  inspection 111, 128, 129, 196, 210
  matching process 112, 117–22, 141
  need for state resources 150
  people with dementia 97
  personalisation 59
  potential 189
  professional boundaries 22
  risk management approach 126–31
  self-employment 113, 195–6
  wellbeing as aim 141
Shared Lives Plus 116, 134
Sheffield, H. 207
short termism 59, 110, 120, 146, 157
Sitch, T. 184, 185
slow food movement 174
slow policy movement 173–5, 176, 215
small-state approach 34, 49, 81
Smith, D. 192
social capital 90, 179, 184
Social Care White Paper 2012 41
social connections 108, 155–7, 176
social franchising 196
social isolation 37, 91, 145, 155
social media 158, 181
social prescribing 99, 185
South London Cares 200
Southern Cross 61, 62